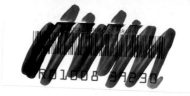
Journey into Personhood

Singular Lives: The Iowa Series in North American Autobiography
Albert E. Stone, Series Editor

Journey into Personhood

by Ruth Cameron Webb

Foreword by Albert E. Stone

UNIVERSITY OF IOWA PRESS IOWA CITY

University of Iowa Press, Iowa City 52242

Copyright © 1994 by the University of Iowa Press

Printed in the United States of America

Design by Karen Copp

Printed on acid-free paper

Library of Congress Cataloging-in-Publication Data

Webb, Ruth Cameron, 1923–

   Journey into personhood / by Ruth Cameron Webb;
   foreword by Albert E. Stone.

       p.   cm.— (Singular lives)

    ISBN 0-87745-470-1, ISBN 0-87745-471-X (pbk.)

    1. Webb, Ruth Cameron, 1923– —Health.

   2. Cerebral palsied—Iowa—Biography. I. Title.

   II. Series.

   RC388.W43   1994

   362.1′96836′0092—dc20

   [B]   94-25881

                                      CIP

01 00 99 98 97 96 95 94 C 5 4 3 2 1

01 00 99 98 97 96 95 94 P 5 4 3 2 1

This book is lovingly dedicated to my parents

and to the Chief Spirit Guide and His many helpers,

who have helped my shuttle weave over and under the warp

of physical disability with a woof of multicolored love.

Contents

Foreword

Albert E. Stone

R uth Webb's *Journey into Personhood*, the ninth volume in Iowa's by now firmly established Singular Lives series, is in several respects its most singular story to date. First of all, hers is a searingly honest account of a woman's development with, through, and beyond cerebral palsy. From her childhood confrontation with often bitter and brutal stereotyping as "a spastic," she has struggled to become a mature, well-educated, independent Christian woman who happens to have c.p. Ruth Webb has, in fact, become her self. Each stage of this universal—and very American—process is convincingly recaptured in the words and strategies used by other successful autobiographers: detailed description and dialogue, dramatic anecdote and poetic metaphor, hot emotion and cool reflection. She thus attains the dual role of a good autobiographer, for she simultaneously authenticates a past shared with others (writes, that is, a memoir) while performing as her present authorial self (and so constructs a confession). The result is a social and psychological document of permanent value to any reader alive to the range and diversity of contemporary American experience and expression.

Some readers, though, may welcome this woman's singular story because they believe it is almost unique, that few disabled Americans have actually written memorable autobiographies. Compared to other marginalized persons and groups, this is so. Social and economic formations controlling the writing, publication, and reception of books have often worked to limit accounts about people who are blind or who have serious disabilities, just as significant numbers of minorities, women, gays and lesbians, prisoners, exiles, and others on the edges have only recently found voices and venues for telling their own intimate stories.

But the relative rarity of *Journey into Personhood* is only partly true. Many readers will remember from schooldays Helen Keller's remarkable memoir, *The Story of My Life*, if not that classic's several sequels. Between 1903 and 1994, there appeared more than a few valuable personal histories about being disabled or afflicted mentally and physically. As the bibliographies of Louis Kaplan and Patricia Addis attest, most of these autobiographies deal with blindness, deafness, cancer, tuberculosis, or polio. Cerebral palsy, with its usual origin in birth injury and its outward manifestations in severe muscular dysfunction, especially spastic movements, blurred speech, and often lifelong use of a wheelchair, is a condition not much welcomed by the reading public. None of those who have cerebral palsy, after all, can report a cure or even a radical cessation of symptoms, though all such narratives may demonstrate that people with cerebral palsy possess brains and creative imaginations. Grace Hoopes's *Out of the Running* (1939), Evelyn Ayrault's *Take One Step* (1963), and Dorothea Waitzmann's *A Special Way of Victory* (1964) are three predecessors (none now in print) of Ruth Webb's life history.

While these narratives (all, significantly, written by women) share common literary themes, none excels Webb's in recording, sometimes in excruciating detail, the inner turmoil people with cerebral palsy go through to win mastery over impaired muscles and voices, rocky social relationships, and insensitive public perceptions. "Some days I cry for hours," Webb confesses. Often she prays for healing not of her physical affliction but of the fear, anger, and frustration that continually exacerbate it. Thus, the explicit aim of *Journey into Personhood* is "to portray the psychological impact of an all-encompassing physical disability on mental and emotional growth." Though she never learns to walk or speak "normally," Ruth Webb celebrates what is in many respects an American success story.

Perhaps the most characteristic personal and cultural trait helping this author to attain, against tremendous odds, a Ph.D. in clinical psychology and a career in counseling and evaluation is her determination. As one educational setting after another proves hostile or inadequate, she persists. High school mastery of English, French, Latin, algebra, and biology is finally accompanied by greater mastery over a still unruly body and fearful mind. With help from some loving teachers and the "crab" (a tripod walker), she conquers her fear of falling in open spaces. "So I walk at age seventeen," she reports with quiet pride. This announcement underscores a crucial somatic difference between her disability and Helen Keller's blindness and deafness. Mobility opens the realms of nature to the Alabama girl, whose whole body, filling the void of eyes and ears, becomes alive to the environment she's able to encounter in run and romp, on pony and bicycle, and in a canoe. Ruth Webb, on the other hand, battles for years to achieve the freedom of a lightweight electric wheelchair. And her academic ambition (since she can read and write more easily than Keller) is steadier. While young Helen learns at Radcliffe that "I am not avaricious for wisdom or knowledge," Ruth surges steadily ahead in her quest, winning a B.A. *cum laude* from Drew, an M.A. at Syracuse, and finally the Ph.D. at the University of Illinois. To cite what

I think is an appropriate parallel, no slave narrative in our literature (even Booker T. Washington's) demonstrates more convincingly the human quality of persistence and the love of literary and academic attainment—goals that can seem "easy" or "normal" to other Americans.

Vital to this success in school and career are two other social circumstances and values often taken for granted. The first is the loving, lasting, sacrificial support of the Webb family—father, mother, aunts, brother. "In my experience, determined parents ultimately win," Ruth remarks of a fellow student's analogous situation. Beyond the domestic circle, too, she finds a succession of friendly mentors and "spirit guides." One of these is Dr. Hann of Syracuse. He inspires her to determine her own pace and progress by deciding her own grade in his courses. At first Ruth gives herself a B. "I'm a slow learner," she tells her teacher, herself, and the reader, "but I won't forget this lesson." Thus armed by trust and responsibility, she redoubles her efforts and finally gives herself an A.

Underlying both family and school experiences is the challenge of independence. This crucial cultural value is complicated at every turn in Ruth Webb's case by the demands of her body and her reliance on others—not just the mother and father who scrimp to give her academic opportunities but also the fellow students and friends who open doors, carry her tray, type her thesis, hug her, and dry her tears. The activity of writing, like her professional work with disabled clients in Wisconsin, Pennsylvania, and Iowa, sharpens this paradoxical balance between leaning on others and fending for herself. As Eudora Welty has observed of independence in her autobiography, *One Writer's Beginnings*, "To grow up is to fight for it, to grow old is to lose it after having possessed it." For one wrestling with cerebral palsy for more than seventy years, this wise aphorism has a special edge. Ruth has had to fight against the very mother who has sacrificed so much for her daughter's survival and success but whose fearful possessiveness must finally be rejected.

This inner struggle gives a poignant power to the later chapters of *Journey into Personhood*. There, a striking feature of Ruth Webb's story emerges as both a pattern of actual experience and a metaphor of self. The interactions of social and psychological awareness and action are represented in the rooms, houses, school buildings, and hospitals she has successively inhabited. Domestic and public spaces thus symbolize growth and obstacle. Again, the contrast with Helen Keller is instructive. While the youthful autobiographer of *The Story of My Life* glories in memories and evocations of woods, fields, lakes, and ocean, condemning the city and the lecture hall, Ruth Webb marks her much longer pilgrimage by the narrow passageway and wide reception hall, the shared dormitory room, the slippery library steps, and the stages she must cross to seal social acceptance and win academic success. These interior spaces are as likely to be seen as threats or traps as refuges for body and spirit. But the urge to live in safety within her own space is finally realized in the home she and her devoted housekeeper, Belinda, buy in Red Wing, Iowa: "For me, owning the 'Little Red House' is an irrefutable mark of personhood." Her elderly mother can now be taken care of by the daughter instead of the other way around. If in the book's last pages the autobiographer writes with real feeling of her new life in a Christian retirement home, this serenity has been dearly purchased by giving care to others *and* by the independence of the giver. "In our own apartment, Belinda and I each have a bedroom and bath, and I have room for my IBM computer and for the remnant of my book collection. The Entrance's automatic doors and convenient curb cuts along four blocks give me the long-wanted freedom to shop in town and to go to church alone," Webb writes. For nondisabled readers who can imagine their own retirement in a nursing home, these low-keyed words resonate with a particular power.

Likewise loaded with personal and wider significance are Ruth Webb's last words above. "To go to church alone" seems to summon up nothing more momentous than a conventional weekly ritual in a small midwestern college town. But in this life story, freedom and worship have from the early pages gone together. The "spirit guides," or supporting presences, presiding over Webb's life are God's messengers, and these are usually churchgoers. Hence *Journey into Personhood* must be read as at base a spiritual autobiography. Neither body, mind, nor social identity is ultimately determinative; this writer's "soul-sense," rather, is the core of her being. A force beyond intervenes periodically to aid and mark the "spastic" actor and unite her to the remembering writer. These spiritual presences and their effects are first heralded in the blanket mentioned in the preface. Though the young Native American weaver can see only the snarls and knots on her blanket's underside, the Great Spirit in heaven shows her the beautiful other side all the world has seen, the side the "spirit guides" have helped her weave into her life's blanket. Baptism, church membership, and enlightened pastors and chaplains represent way stations of a spiritual pilgrimage marked from beginning to end by her anguished yet hopeful question: Will I ever be able to thank God for my disability?

A decisive step forward on this spiritual journey occurs at Camps Farthest Out in upstate New York. There, Carola, a beautiful dancer, teaches Ruth by loving her for who she is. "Ruth dear, don't worry about *doing*," she urges, "just *be*." Carola's faith, augmented by that of others at CFO, opens the way to a key experience, one that characteristically takes place inside a building. While a famous evangelist is preaching in the camp chapel, "suddenly, a strong wind starts from the narthex and sweeps through the Norman-style church with a mighty Pentecostal surge. That night there is no doubt in any one's mind that we have been visited by the Holy Spirit."

Nevertheless, spirit guides and ecstatic moments cannot displace the equally vivid moments of loneliness, fear, and anger that accompany every stage of Ruth Webb's journey. Only by revisiting her whole life in the process of writing her autobiography has she come to terms with her body and mind and thereby claimed, temporarily at least, a measure of serene assurance of God's love. "I now realize my ongoing journey into personhood has led me along the path of faith," she concludes. "My search for integrity as a person has not only brought yearned-for opportunities to give and receive love. In that giving and receiving, my grandfather's prediction has come true. I have come to know the Son of the Great Spirit." In that process, she has woven her own blanket with words that reflect both the underside of snarls and knots in her turbulent experience and the beautiful design of loving colors on the other side of self.

Prologue

Once my grandfather, whom I adored, told this story to me as I sat on his lap.

Many, many moons ago, there lived a young Native American girl who spent her days weaving blankets. Her blankets were so beautiful that many warriors came to her wigwam and asked her to join their campfires. She always looked at the blanket which was on her loom and, seeing only the knots and snarls of the underside, hung her head in shame and declined the fine offers.

Winters and summers came and went, and the girl became a wrinkled and bent old woman. Still she persisted in weaving the blankets for which she was famous. Never did she look at the upper side of the blankets when she took them off her loom. She tossed them in a heap in a corner, and their beauty was seen only by those who took them home and used them to keep warm. The old woman continued to look at only the knots and snarls of each blanket's underside, the only side she could see when the blanket was on the loom.

The time finally came for the old woman to go to the wigwam of the Great Spirit. When she reached the entrance, it was the Great Spirit who admitted her into a huge circular dwelling. On its walls hung the most colorful and beautiful blankets she had ever seen.

Holding a finger to his lips for silence, the Great Spirit led the old woman over to the most gorgeous blanket of all. Bright reds and blues were skillfully blended into an amazingly complex pattern. Silently the Great Spirit folded back a corner of the marvelous blanket.

The old one gasped. For there she saw her own knots and snarls on the underside of the prized blanket. The knots and snarls underlay a work of great beauty. Only now, when her life's weaving was finished, could she behold the intricate pattern held together by the knots and snarls of her days.

(Here my beloved grandfather added his own ending to the Indian legend.)

The Great Spirit bent low and whispered in the old one's ear. "I allowed you to make those knots on the underside of your blanket so they would tie together the many strands—beautiful as well as ugly—which weave through your life's pattern."

The idea of the self begins to form very early from the attitudes of family and friends surrounding the infant. Acceptance and rejection by these important people merge into the child's self-image.

As a young girl (me!) gains motor and cognitive control of herself, she increasingly participates in family and community affairs. The youngster's sense of self-esteem develops when the family attitudes foster her confidence that she can ably do the tasks given to her. The growing person feels proud to be considered a contributing and trustworthy member of the family and begins to form a sense of her own worth and integrity. As she grows, her self-image expands and shrinks many times as she is challenged by triumphs and tragedies on her journey into personhood.

But what of the young girl who is so physically disabled from birth that she never learns to walk and talk normally? How does she develop a self-picture of worth and integrity? How do the deeds and attitudes of family, friends, teachers, and scoffers affect the ways in which this future adult copes with the traumatic situations her disability will invariably bring her? What happens when she experiences direction from the "Chief Spirit Guide"?

Journey into Personhood relates how people and events crossed my path at the right times and in the right ways and combined to help me cope with cerebral palsy and become a contributing person.

My purpose in telling my story is to portray the psychological impact of an all-encompassing physical disability on mental and emotional growth. Inextricably woven through this story are the many times I have been helped by both human and heavenly spirit guides. Without their aid, this book would not have been written.

As the motif for this book, I have selected the Native American story about the weaver because it seems that only in looking back do the knots and snarls in one's life tapestry assume their real meaning. There comes a time when hurts and insults—the knots—lose their sting and we are reconciled to the lessons they have taught. When we accept responsibility for the tangles as well as the bright threads in our blankets, we are able to appreciate the beauty of our total pattern. It takes much living to gain this view, and then only in snatches do we see the true patterns we have made.

Because my life has been so occupied with lessening the effects of a birth injury, other aspects of my existence have often been neglected. The Great Spirit's invitation to the old weaver reminds me that in the end, the whole pattern, rather than the tangles in my woof, will most truly reflect my finished fabric.

I hope that *Journey into Personhood* will prompt readers to look beyond the abnormal movements and sounds of cerebral palsy and to see the individual striving to be a whole person.

My story began June 1, 1923, when I was born in an army hospital at Fort Shafter in Hawaii. My father, William Henry Webb, was a second lieutenant in the Coast Artillery Corps of the United States Army.

My mother, Ruth Cameron Webb, came from upstate New York. She had a teaching certificate from Geneseo Normal School and taught first grade for several years. Mother was a gifted manager and salesperson who energetically pursued badly needed extra cash for her family by selling children's books door to door.

My brother, David, was born in 1926 and was my constant companion before I left home for boarding school at the age of twelve. He has led a productive life as a banker, town official, and lawyer and is a much-loved advisor for his sister, wife, four daughters, and four granddaughters as well as for his community.

My grandparents, Charles and Julia Webb, met at Simpson College near Des Moines and raised their children—Ethel, William, and Louise—on a farm in rural Iowa. Aunt Ethel was a Ph.D. candidate when she married Harold U. Faulkner, a well-known Smith College professor and author of several American history textbooks.

My family's names and those of the Rev. Joseph P. Bishop, Glenn Clark, Dr. Frank Lankard, Dr. Frank Laubach, Dr. James A. McClintock, Professor Wilga Rivers, the Rev. Chet Simmons, Alice Shipley, Susan Stedman, the Rev. Tommy Tyson, and Carola Bell Williams are real. I have changed other names to avoid offending or embarrassing individuals who touched my life.

I acknowledge with great appreciation the moral and editorial support given by Dr. Bishop, Pat Cushing, and Ted Mokricky and the helpful comments of my brother, David, and sister-in-law, Frances Webb. Invaluable direction was also given by Leedice Kissane and Paula V. Smith. The steadfast typing of my scribes, Joseph Cushing, Stephanie Ford, Melissa Bolen, and Becky Franklin, enabled this book to be born.

Journey into Personhood

1

Prejourney Memories

This chapter presents a panorama of scenes from my early childhood, which set the stage for my journey into personhood. These pictures from the gallery of my memories represent formative events I have recalled or heard from others. They seem to cast illuminating glances on my lifelong struggle to gain personhood, i.e., integrity, in my own eyes as well as in the eyes of others.

I was prepared for my journey by a loving family, which included my parents, my baby brother, my grandparents, and two aunts. Each person aided my development in a unique way and gave me the desire to become a contributing citizen. I have collected memory pictures from my early childhood and hung them in an imaginary gallery of memories. I invite you, my reader, to accompany me on a trip to view these prejourney memories.

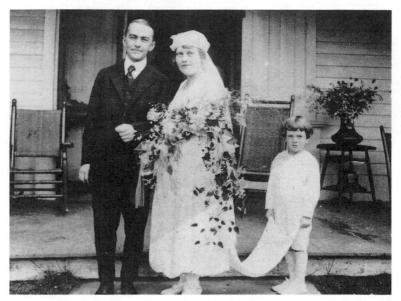

Ruth Gray Cameron and William Henry Webb on their wedding day, June 22, 1921

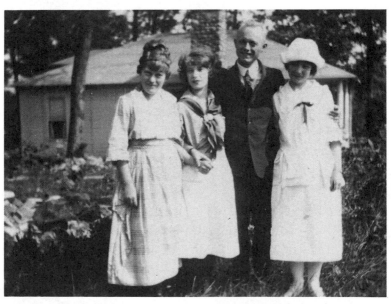

Grandpa Charles and Nan, Julia Webb (at right), with daughters Louise (left) and Ethel

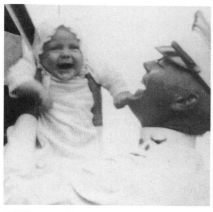

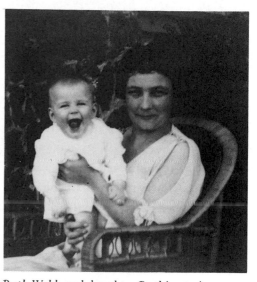

William Webb and daughter Ruthie at four months

Ruth Webb and daughter Ruthie at nine months

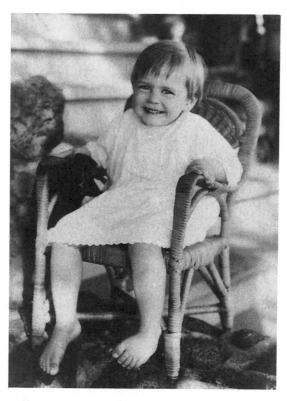

Ruthie at three years

The pictures are not in strict chronological order but are grouped in clusters centering around persons and events making physical and psychological impacts on me. Through backward glances at these scenes, I explore the development of my self-concept and the origin of my sense of integrity.

The inscription accompanying each cluster and scene describes its remembered significance for my journey into personhood. At occasional intervals in the gallery, I present word portraits of the significant people of my early years.

FIRST CLUSTER OF MEMORIES: DEVELOPING A SPASTIC IDENTITY

Early memories of physical examinations and acting-out play have traumatic effects upon me as a young child.

Birthing My Spastic Identity

At the edge of my early memory, I am about three years old. I hear . . .

"Undress her, please!"

Mommy, Daddy, and I are sitting beside a big desk in a strange room. Daddy is talking to a man who wears a white coat.

Suddenly Mommy leans me forward on her lap and unbuttons my dress. She takes off my dress and lays me on a cold table to take off my panties. I cry as she unlaces one high-top shoe. Daddy undresses my other foot.

"Stop crying! Behave like a big girl," Mommy says sternly. "Dr. Hatt won't hurt you."

The doctor bends over me and lifts first one leg and then the other high in the air. I cry and scream loudly. He rolls me over and runs his fingers up and down my back. I shiver and cry again.

After the doctor finishes with me, Mommy dresses me and holds me on her lap again. I stop crying.

"Dr. Hatt, what is wrong with Ruthie?" Daddy asks the doctor.

"How long did you say her birth was?" the doctor asks.

"Twenty-nine hours," Mommy replies.

"When did you notice she was handicapped?"

"At six months, when she didn't sit up without support," Mommy answers.

"Were there any other signs that something was wrong?" the doctor probes. "Any crying spells?"

"Even now there are nights when we can't stop her crying," Daddy answers. "She draws her legs up like she's in pain."

Dr. Hatt sighs. "Lt. and Mrs. Webb," he says, looking at me. "Ruth's having leg spasms when she cries like that. The areas in the brain which control her limb movements were damaged because she didn't receive enough oxygen during her long birth. Ruth is now a spastic child."

"Is she normal mentally?" queries Mommy anxiously.

"She seems a healthy child with normal reactions to strangers," affirms the doctor. "I think she has at least average intelligence."

"You are the first of many doctors to tell us what is wrong with Ruthie. Will she ever walk—and talk?" Daddy finally asks.

"Your daughter will probably run before she is twelve years old, and she should talk in a couple of years."

"Dr. Hatt, what can we do to help her walk and talk?" asked Mommy.

"Let her move on her own as much as possible. Talk to her and encourage her to communicate her needs. She'll do fine."

Word Portrait

Aunt Louise, Daddy's younger sister, has blond hair and blue eyes and is always well groomed. She is very outspoken, with strong opinions about how little girls should dress and say please and thank-you. Aunt Louise is kind and thoughtful and often takes me home. She loves dogs and flowers.

Acting Out My Spastic Identity

Aunt Louise comes upon five-year-old me undressing the doll she has just given me.

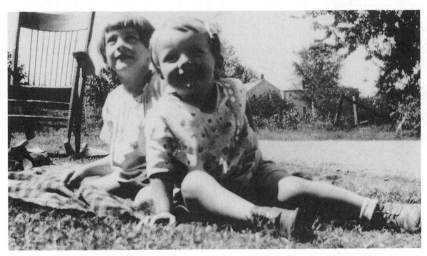

Ruthie at five years with two-year-old Budge

"Ruthie, why, for heaven's sake, do you insist on taking off the pretty clothes of every new doll?" she asks.

"Oh," I say, "I have to! The doctor's going to 'xamine her 'cause she's a spastic!"

Owning My Spastic Identity

"Why can't you walk?" asked one boy. "You talk funny!"

"Are you Chinese?" asks a tall girl.

Everyone laughs and the ice is broken. This is my introduction to classmates in a first grade for army-post children.

I turn red with embarrassment. Then I remember how Mommy has told me to answer such questions, and I explain: "I can't walk yet because I was hurt when I was a baby, but I'm going to walk some day. And I'm not Chinese, but I talk my own way. If you listen real hard, you'll understand me."

Enlarging the Scope of My Spastic Identity

I tell Mommy, "I must have a white dress! I am going to be in a parade with my class."

She looks at me sadly. "No, Ruthie," she says. "You can't be in the parade. You can't walk!"

These words hit me with a thud.

"Can't walk!" I think. "Why can't someone push my chair?"

Realizing I Have a Communication Gap

The boy on my left whispers, "I like ice cream."

I whisper to the boy on my other side, "I like ice cream."

He turns red and turns to his pal next to him and giggles.

I flush a deep red and say aloud, "He can't understand me."

Meeting Rejection Because of My Identity

A lady opens the door of the tourist home, and giving me a suspicious look, she asks Mommy in a sharp tone, "What is wrong with your child? Is she retarded?"

"No," explains Mommy. "Ruthie is spastic, but she's as bright as any child!"

"Humph! She looks strange to me. I don't want her in my house!" With this declaration, the woman slams the door.

Mommy looks at me and then at Daddy, who is balancing me.

"Well," she says slowly, "I guess we don't want to stay in her house either."

Then, looking straight at me, she continues: "Ruthie, there will always be people who don't understand you. But then, there will always be those who love you."

I whisper to myself. "Why doesn't this lady want me around? Why do some grown-ups say I'm smarter than I am? Why can't they take me for what I am, a ten-year-old girl who can't walk?"

SECOND CLUSTER OF MEMORIES: TRYING TO OVERCOME
MY SPASTIC IDENTITY

In our Fort Banks home, I am pretty much the center of a small universe. The weekly schedule revolves around our trips to the muscle-training clinic in Boston and my therapist's visits in our home.

Training Righty as well as Lefty

"You say Ruthie is four years old. She's so tiny!" marvels Miss Russo, a young therapist from the Boston clinic to my mother. "She's starting training none too soon."

Twice a week I lie on the dining room table and let this person with the short dark hair and pretty brown eyes bend first one knee and then the other in reciprocal fashion. Then she raises my arms above my head and bends and straightens my elbows, wrists, and fingers.

While she moves my limbs, Miss Russo says, "Ruthie, this is Lefty, your good foot, and here is Lefty, your good hand. Your lazy hand and foot I call Righty Hand and Righty Foot."

When she finishes with my exercises, she says in her sweet voice, "Now Dearie, let's relax you with a good rubdown!"

As Miss Russo massages, I smile contentedly. When she says good-by, I hug her.

Being Frustrated by Impossible Demands

"Just lean forward, Ruth. The hanging saddle will move when you put all your weight on one foot and lean forward. Try hard!"

Miss Patton is chief therapist at the Boston Muscle-Training Clinic. Her eyes flash with anger and her voice rises.

I lean forward and push with both hands in an all-out effort to move the hanging saddle, a canvas bag, with two holes for my legs, which hangs from a hook in a metal groove in the ceiling.

Miss Patton scolds and I cry angry tears of frustration. I tremble with fear.

I try again and again, but I never lean forward enough to make the saddle move.

Resisting Walking Practice (Much Later)

"Mommy, I don't want to walk now. I want to read how Nancy Drew solves another mystery."

Tears stream down Mommy's face. "Ruthie, don't you know how important your learning to walk is? Great things will happen when you walk. You may even go to college and earn your own living. And if you never walk, I don't know what will happen to you! Please walk for me, or practice with the parallel bars Daddy made for you."

"Mommy," I cry, "I'll practice walking with you. Stay right behind me. I'm so scared of big, empty rooms."

She stands behind me while I take twenty-five steps.

Feeling Alone on Life's Railroad

"Mommy! Daddy! Come quick!" I cry from my bed. "I'm on that flatcar again. Everything is black around me. The car is rolling forward on two white tracks that stretch to the horizon. It is going faster and faster. I'm passing you, Daddy, and Budge. I will never see you again."

"Sweetie," says Mommy, bending over me. "You've had a bad dream again. Don't be afraid. You'll never be alone. Daddy and I won't let you ride away from us."

Singing with Peers

In a speech therapy group for young children, the teacher suddenly stops playing the piano, turns to me, and says quietly, "Ruth, did I hear you singing 'Mary Had a Little Lamb'? I am very proud of you!"

Smiling, I nod my head, "Yes!"

Word Portrait

Mommy has a slight build and is full of nervous energy. She is determined to overcome my handicap with daily training. She makes me stick to her routine. Mommy certainly is queen of my small universe.

Drilling My Feeding and Dressing Skills

"Ruthie," says Mommy, taking my hand. "Here is a silver spoon with the handle made into a loop. Stick your fingers in the loop and grasp it tightly. Now dip the spoon in the applesauce and take it to your mouth. Good! You'll feed yourself before you know it.

"While you're eating, remember to sit up straight, Ruthie. Keep your mouth closed and don't drool," reminds my mother. "And tomorrow I will show you how to put your arms in your sleeves before drawing your dress over your head."

Practicing Speech at Home

"Put your lips together and blow to say *F*. Try again. You made a good *F* that time!"

Mommy is trying very hard to get me to talk at home. Every evening she makes me practice saying *F*, *V*, *L*, and *S*. I turn to grab my doll.

Mommy says, "Oh, so you're tired of practicing sounds. Now we will try some tongue exercises."

She picks up a bath towel and grasps my tongue with it. She pulls it hard. Ugh! The rough towel sends shivers down my back and my stretched tongue hurts.

"We will practice every morning until you learn to talk," declares Mommy. "I am determined to have you talking by the time you are four years old."

Toilet Training with Mommy

"Why didn't you tell me you had to go before I put you in your high chair? You must let me know before you wet yourself!" cries Mommy. "You are almost ten years old, and it's time for you to stop wetting yourself."

"I'm hungry. I want to eat," I say, hanging my head.

Mommy answers, "Whenever you delay going to the bathroom, your pants get wet and a puddle always appears under your chair. What am I going to do with you?"

THIRD CLUSTER OF MEMORIES: DEVELOPING PERSISTENCE

This picture recalls my first adventure on my own. Getting up the hill shows me that persistence leads to results.

Climbing on My Own

I am on the edge of the gently sloping hill beside our house.

Tall grass covers the hill by our house, and I often crawl on my knees to the rim of the hill to look at the shallow gully below.

One day I lean too far over the edge of this miniprecipice, and down I go, rolling over and over, until I reach the bottom. I quickly realize that it's up to me to get up the hill because there is no one around to call for help.

I try to climb back up on the slippery grass. I move my knees one, two, three times. My left knee slides back while I'm pulling the right one up. I get tired and barely move my left knee. It stays put. I then inch my right knee up. It stays put too. In this way, I move slowly up the hill, inch by inch. When I finally reach the top, I look up at the sky.

I laugh and say out loud, "I can roll down the hill whenever I want. I can have my own fun!"

FOURTH CLUSTER OF MEMORIES: MY FIRST GREAT GOAL

Learning to walk was the first goal presented to me by my parents. Wonderful things would happen with this achievement—school, college, a job. I would even be like other kids.

At first, I do not see a need to restrict my present mobility for the promise of an ability to walk in the future.

Forbidding Crawling

"If you want Ruth to walk, don't ever let her crawl on her knees again. Further crawling will leave her knees permanently bent, and then she'll never walk." So saying, Miss Patton leaves me in tearful despair.

Mommy puts her arm around me. I sob, "I can't crawl around the yard anymore. No more rolling down my hill. I can't even move from room to room at home!"

Mommy whispers softly, "Daddy and I will help you walk everywhere you want to go. Let me show you how. Stand on your feet and I will hold your shoulders. Now, put Lefty forward and then Righty, and lean on them as you step. See, you can do it. Daddy and I will always be with you to help you walk."

Adjusting to Rules

"Ruthie, have you been on your knees again? You won't ever walk that way. I want you to walk and run like other girls."

I blush and hang my head. I mutter, "If I can't crawl, I can't make any more petunia meringue mud pies."

Mommy hugs me and says, "You can make mud pies with your knees straight. When you do, use oak leaves for your meringue, not my petunias. Dig with Righty, as well as with Lefty."

Pulling Up to Stand

I am alone in the kitchen and have just pulled myself up to stand by the sink. Mommy enters, throws her arms around me, and exclaims, "Ruthie, you got to your feet by yourself. I'm proud of you. Keep trying and I know you'll walk some day. I so want you to walk!"

Just then Daddy creeps up behind me and throws his arms around me, proclaiming loudly, "I've got ya! My standing-up girl!"

Expressing a Deep Wish

"Here is the doll you wanted so much," says Mommy, handing me a doll which is two feet tall.

"Does she really walk and talk like the ad said?" I ask.

"Hold her up and see what she does," advises Mommy.

I try hard to make the doll walk, but it crumples up and falls down whenever I let go. I tell Mommy, "I thought the newspaper said she could walk and talk. I wanted her because I thought she could teach me to walk."

I begin to cry. Mommy hugs me and says, "You are seven years old, and it's time for you to learn that not everything the newspaper says is true."

I reply, "Well, I'm going to call her Walky-Talky. Maybe someday we will both walk and talk."

FIFTH CLUSTER OF MEMORIES: BUDGE

In my early years, my little brother, David, whom I call Budge, is my constant playmate. He is three years younger than me and is the chief peer with whom I play and fight, lead and follow, manipulate and love.

Word Portrait

Budge is a small, sturdy fellow with blue eyes and blond hair. He greatly enjoys winning arguments with his undisputable statements. He facilitates my participation in our joint play.

Witnessing My Brother's First Walk

I am in the playroom with Budge. I hear him giggle and look up from my doll to see him taking his first steps, wobbling some, but walking clear across the room. I call Mommy, who comes running. She kneels down and hugs Budge, saying, "Ruthie, I hope you walk soon." I say, "Me, too!"

Learning Not to Tell about Bumps

Five-year-old Budge is pushing his eight-year-old sister around the Antlers, my grandmother's inn in the Pocono Mountains. I am in my reed wheelchair, which is almost too big for Budge to push over bumpy ground. I often land on the ground, but I am never really hurt. I get on my knees, grab the arm rests, pull to a stand, and sit down again. Then we continue on our way.

I warn Budge, "Don't tell Mommy I fell. She won't let you push me anymore!"

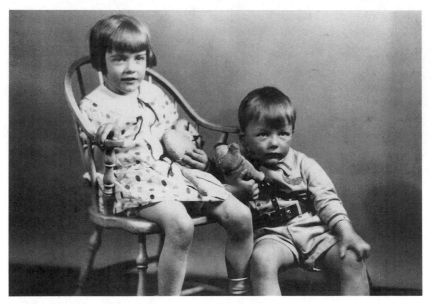

Ruthie at eight years with five-year-old Budge

SIXTH CLUSTER OF MEMORIES: PARTICIPATING IN FAMILY LOVE AND FUN

Affectionate recognition for my small accomplishments and funny antics and special attention from Nan and Grandpa make me truly feel a participant in family affairs.

Word Portrait

Daddy has a medium build with blond hair and blue eyes. He laughs often, especially when he is teasing. He is always ready to play, repair household fixtures, or make equipment for his daughter. He helps Mommy with household chores. He is usually kind and patient but shows a temper when repeatedly frustrated. He is always a good companion, even if he is often silent.

Fun with My Daddy

Daddy and I are sitting at the big dining room table, looking at my baby pictures in the family album, which is so carefully kept by Mommy. Daddy points to a large snapshot. "Look, Ruthie. There you are, sitting on your sled in the snow. You were just three years old when I nailed that three-sided wooden box to your sled to support your back and sides. You are laughing and having fun in the snow." Daddy turns the page. "See this picture. You are sitting on your first tricycle and I am standing right behind you. You sure are enjoying doing the same things as other kids."

Taking Does Not Always Mean Keeping

Daddy and three-year-old me are in a department store. As I am facing backward over his shoulder, he doesn't see me reach with Lefty for a very attractive doll, dressed in pink and white.

"A baby!" I whisper. "Now I'll have a baby like Mommy does!"

Daddy turns and sees the large baby doll in my arms. "We have to return the doll," he tells me, despite my loud protests. "The doll isn't yours. It belongs to the store!"

Then Daddy declares, "From now on, I'm calling you Little Pili-kia. That word means *trouble* in Hawaiian."

Waiting Brings Tears

"Where can Daddy be? He's ten minutes late. The pool closes at five o'clock. I won't get my three laps around the pool, and Private Luke won't like that!"

My chest tightens, and tears course down my cheeks. Mommy stops in the door and says sharply, "Stop crying, Ruthie! You're a big girl!"

Her words make me cry more. The harder I try to stop, the tighter my chest becomes and the longer I cry.

Making Daddy Cross

"Stop crying, Ruthie! I don't know what you want. You say you want oatmeal, and when you have it, you push it aside and demand a boiled egg. I take you for a ride in the car. You cry to come home.

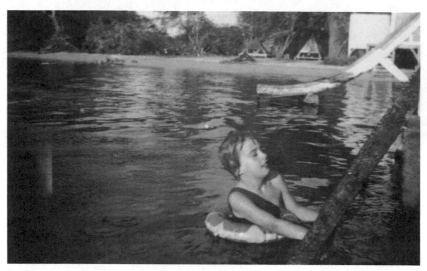

Ruthie in pool at Ft. Kamehameha on the island of Oahu, 1932

We got back here an hour ago and you're still weeping! Now you want a car ride again.

"I'm going to turn you over my knee, spank you, and put you in bed. That is the only way I know to stop this crying!" Daddy declares.

He turns me bottom up and gives me three whacks with an open hand. Then he carries me to my bed and stays outside my room until my crying subsides.

Swinging with Daddy

Budge and I are in the back yard of the Antlers. On a branch of a big oak, Daddy has hung a rope swing. Budge is swinging when Daddy walks over to us.

"Ruthie, would you like to try swinging?"

"Yes!" I squeal.

"Sonny, will you let your sister have a turn on the swing?"

Daddy seats me and makes each of my hands grasp a rope. My legs stiffen out in front of me. Righty slips from the rope and Daddy puts it back, giving me a little shove. The ground fades away and

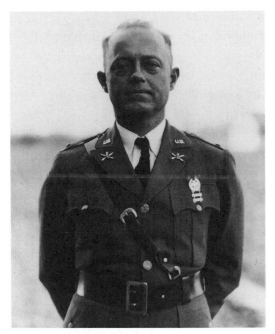

William Webb, 1933

then comes back. I'm having fun. I squeal with delight as I go higher and higher.

"Hold on tight!" warns Daddy, as I lean too far back and almost fall.

I cry, "I am flying like a bird! I am swinging just like any other kid!"

Word Portrait

Nan, my Grandma Webb, is a big lady with a reddish gray bun behind her head. She is a great cook and hardly ever uses a recipe for her delicious soups, casseroles, and desserts. Kind and generous, she is always telling me stories and making dresses for me.

Helping Nan Shuck Corn

I am in Nan's kitchen when Daddy brings in a basket of freshly picked corn.

"Let me shuck the corn!" I exclaim.

Nan looks dubious. "Can you shuck all that corn before dinner?"

"Please let me try," I urge.

Nan gives me two baskets for the shucked ears and for the corn leaves. She puts a pile of unshucked cobs within Lefty's reach and says, "Ruthie, go to it!"

I hold an ear with Righty, pull the shucks off with Lefty, and throw them in the leaves basket. I brush the silk off with my fingers and lay the undressed ear on the table. By the time I shuck five ears, I begin to work faster.

When I finally put the last ear on the table, I squeal with delight, "Nan, I shucked every ear of corn for dinner!"

Nan smiles, "You sure did, and with fifteen minutes to spare! You are a great help."

I reply, "Nan, you really needed me to shuck corn. I'm glad I helped you. I love you!"

Word Portrait

A tall, lanky gentleman with black vest, coat, and blue tie, a storyteller and a game player (but not on Sundays), and a deeply committed Christian with an unshakable faith in Jesus Christ— this was my grandfather.

Learning about Jesus from Grandpa

Grandpa and I are in the cemetery of a little white church. Pointing to several white gravestones, Grandpa asserts, "These people are only sleeping. They will wake up when Jesus comes back."

"Grandpa, will I get to see Jesus?" I ask.

He looks at me and smiles. "Well, Ruthie, you just may see Him. You are only eight years old. He may come tomorrow, and He will surely come in your lifetime. Remember He will always be with you."

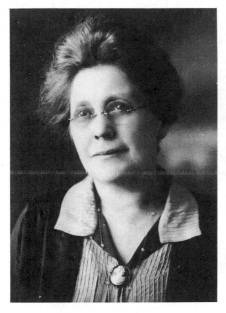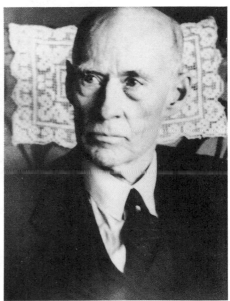

Nan and Grandpa Charles, c. 1933

Believing but Not Understanding Salvation

"Everything the Bible says is true. It tells us we are saved through Christ's death on the cross. You have to believe this to gain salvation. There is no other way," declares Grandpa.

"Grandpa, I don't know what salvation is but it must be very important if you say so."

Wishing to See Jesus

Grandpa and I are spending the night in the bungalow, a white frame cottage in Nan's pine grove.

"What bedroom do you want to sleep in?" Grandpa asks.

"The front bedroom. I like to look up through the rafters."

When I am in bed, I say, "Grandpa, tell me about Jesus."

"Do you want to hear about the boy they let down through the roof so that Jesus could heal him?"

I nod my head. When he finishes the tale, I murmur, "I wish Jesus would come down through the rafters this very night."

Denying That My Handicap Is "Error" (Much Later)

Every Sunday morning, Mother drives Budge and me into the city of Honolulu to attend the Christian Science Sunday School in hopes that its teachings might heal my cerebral palsy.

"If my handicap is not real, why can't I walk and talk like other girls?" I ask Miss Winters, my revered Sunday School teacher.

"Ruth, in the beginning, God created everything perfect. So handicaps are not real. They are 'error,' or mistaken ideas, in your mind. If you can believe that your handicap is 'error,' you will be healed," asserts Miss Winters.

As my teacher turns to another student, I mutter softly, "I can't ever be healed through prayer, but I do wish I could walk."

SEVENTH CLUSTER OF MEMORIES: LEARNING THE THREE R'S

My mother is a teacher and begins my education at home. With the exception of my brief attendance at a private first grade, she teaches me from the first grade through the fifth grade. Then I enjoy attending the sixth grade in public school.

Learning to Read

Mother and I are sitting before a wooden easel in the kitchen. She points to an alphabet chart with the word *at* printed in its right margin.

"Ruthie, remember that the letter *b* says 'Ba,' as in banana. Now I'm going to add the word family 'at' to *b*, and what word do we have? See, we have made the word bat. Now, let's see how many words you can make with the 'at' family."

Printing My Name

I draw a straight mark between two blue lines on my paper. Then I make a circle and attach it to my straight mark. Finally I draw a slanting mark down to the blue line.

Lefty is tired and sweaty, but I have made an *R*. I quickly make

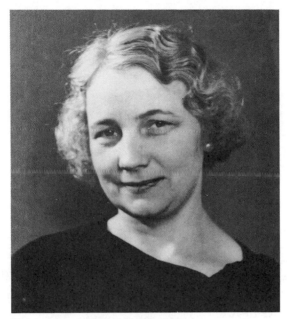

Teacher-mother Ruth Webb, 1933

a cuplike *U*, a straight line with a cross mark for a *T*, and finally an *H*. My name, RUTH, stares up at me.

Learning at Home (Much Later)

"Here is today's sentence for you and Budge to copy ten times. It reads, 'I am learning to write by practicing good penmanship.' When your Lefty gets tired and sweaty, rest it awhile and recite the three times table."

As Mommy leaves to go shopping, she points to some books on my desk. "I got these from the library yesterday. When you finish your writing and math assignments, Ruthie, you may read about your favorite hero, Abraham Lincoln, while Budge gets acquainted with Johnny Appleseed."

EIGHTH CLUSTER OF MEMORIES: AWAKENING A STRONG DESIRE

At an early age, I know that I am left out of many family activities because of my physical handicap. My Aunt Ethel is the one who helps me combat the feeling of rejection by giving me hope that I will someday be able to help people.

Word Portrait

A plump lady of medium stature, Aunt Ethel is adamant that every step in any task she undertakes be completed. For example, every food parcel for a picnic must be wrapped in waxed paper and held in place with strong rubber bands. Despite her very practical nature, my aunt is a liberal thinker and a builder of dreams.

Planting Ambitious Seeds

"Would you like to go to a boarding school?" Aunt Ethel asks.

"A real boarding school? Where I live away from home?"

"Yes!" says Aunt Ethel emphatically. "There's a boarding school near Boston for physically handicapped children. Are you interested?" queries my aunt.

She continues, "Ruthie, if you study hard, someday you may go to college. Who knows? You may even earn your own living!"

"Oh, Aunt Ethel," I cry. "Do you really think that someday I will have a job where I help others?"

So ends the gallery of my early memories. They form the backdrop for the struggles, defeats, and victories which follow in the next chapters.

2

Painful First Steps

"Opportunities are opening up for handicapped people. By the time you grow up, there'll be an important job for you, I'm sure!" my Aunt Ethel concludes her heart-to-heart conversation with me. "I will talk to your parents about sending you to a boarding school."

It is 1935 and I am twelve when Aunt Ethel finally persuades Mommy to send me to the New England Institute for Learning (NEIL), a boarding school for disabled children near Boston, Massachusetts. Daddy is strangely silent in the matter, but when I insist that he voice an opinion, he hugs me and says, "It's your decision, Pilikia. You are old enough to have a say in your future."

This decision is not reached until ten days before Labor Day, and so there is a flurry of preparations. Daddy and I shop for my first low shoes while Mommy and Nan make me four new dresses. Grandpa prints name tapes for all my clothes, and Nan sews them on. During this busy week, Aunt Ethel's prediction that I will some-day have a job rings in my ears, and I can hardly sleep at night. I am going to a "regular school."

The great day comes at last. We meet Aunt Ethel in Boston and go on to Worcester. While riding in the back seat with Mommy, I resolve not to be called Ruthie any longer. Henceforth, I am Ruth. I'm going to call Mommy "Mother" and Daddy "Dad." I announce this decision, and Dad looks back at Mother.

"Our little girl is growing up," Dad says to Mother.

Mother hugs me. "I'll miss you!" she whispers.

"That's the administration building," declares Aunt Ethel. "We go in there."

After Dad parks the car, he tells me, "Pilikia, I have something to tell you. As a new student, you will stay in the infirmary a week or so to make sure you don't have any contagious disease. Then you will move to a girls' cottage where you will have friends your own age."

I am getting uneasy; my stomach is churning. Dad walks me in to a long hall with shiny, slippery stone floors. A man with long leg braces greets us and calls Miss Knight, the school principal.

We sit down in the large waiting room with blue overstuffed chairs. A tall, big-framed lady enters with her hand outstretched. She says softly, "I'm Margaret Knight."

After shaking hands with each of us, Miss Knight sits near me and asks, "Ruth, what grade are you in?"

"Seventh," I reply proudly.

"Oh dear! My seventh grade is really a big class this year."

"Perhaps Ruth can go into the sixth grade," suggests Aunt Ethel.

I glare at her angrily. I have finished the sixth grade.

Miss Knight says hastily, "I think there is room for one more in the class. Don't worry, Ruth. You'll be in my seventh grade."

When the time comes for my family to leave, the lump in my throat grows to gigantic proportions. Mother hugs me and turns quickly away but not before I see the tears streaming down her cheeks.

Aunt Ethel pats my shoulder and says, "Ruthie, I know you'll do your best in school. It won't be long before you move to a cottage."

Dad thumps me on the back and says, "Be good and don't take any wooden nickels!" He holds me close for a moment. "Try hard, Little Pilikia," he whispers. Then he leaves the room very quickly.

I start to cry.

Just then a red haired nurse wearing a blue dress, white apron, and a Dutch cap and pushing an enormous wicker wheelchair enters the room.

"This is Miss Bartlett," says Miss Knight.

"Hello, Ruth Webb. I'm going to take you to the Smyth Infirmary, where we'll learn all about you. Can you get into this wheelchair?"

I nod my head yes and pull myself up to stand, turn around, and sit down. Miss Bartlett then wheels the chair rapidly out the door of the administration building and turns left along a covered walk.

We enter a dingy hall, take the elevator up to the second floor, and go into a long ward with ten beds on each side.

"Ruth, this is your bed," she says, pointing to the second bed on the left side. "Here are your ward mates, Anne, Sally, and Mary. You are all new patients."

I react to the term *patients*. I think, Aren't we students?

"Hi!" Sally smiles. "I have osteoporosis in my hips. I've been here three days. They won't let me go outside yet."

"They won't let us go out till the doctor sees us," adds Mary. "I'm blind and I can't see anything. I've been here almost a week. I'm really bored!"

Anne says nothing but points to her shriveled foot. Tears run down her cheeks.

What have I gotten into? I think.

"Now, now," chides Miss Bartlett. "Things aren't that bad. I hear there'll be a band concert Monday. I'm sure Dr. White will see you before that."

Supper comes at five o'clock. It consists of creamed dried beef on a half-baked potato, canned string beans, milk, and canned peaches for dessert. Ugh! I push the tray away in disgust. Is this all they have to eat at boarding school?

"Don't you like your supper?" asks Miss Bartlett solicitously. "Would you like some ice cream?"

Responding to the clamor of yes from all of us, Miss Bartlett fetches four deep soup bowls, brimming over with vanilla ice cream.

"This will satisfy your hunger." She smiles as we gobble up the ice cream.

All this time I am sitting in a huge wicker wheelchair. My feet become numb from lack of support. I ask timidly, "Miss Bartlett, may I sit in another chair? Please."

"Of course, you may, Ruth. I'll see if we have one your size." She hurries away and returns with a small maple-colored wooden chair with big wheels in front and small swivel wheels in back.

When I am seated in the small chair, Miss Bartlett says, "Now Ruth, take hold of the wheel handles and move the chair."

Lefty turns the metal handle easily, but Righty has trouble gripping and then letting go. The chair moves in circles to the right because I can only push with my left hand.

Then a bright idea strikes me. Why not move forward by stepping with my feet while sitting in the chair? I place my left foot forward and pull at the floor, then I move my right foot and repeat the process.

It works, and the chair moves ahead.

Miss Bartlett beams. "It took five minutes for you to learn to move your chair. I expect great things of you!"

Then she disappears for a moment and returns with a long white canvas strap, which she puts around my waist and then ties in back of my wheelchair.

"There, now, Ruth, you can move all you want and you won't fall out."

"No! No!" I cry. "I don't need to be tied in. I never fall out."

But in spite of my tearful protests, Miss Bartlett does not remove the shame-provoking strap. It is a week before I can look at it without being angry. Eventually I learn to lean on the strap when moving my chair forward with my feet.

Later that evening Miss Bartlett says, "Ruth, it's time for your bath. All new patients get baths the first night they are here."

Miss Bartlett takes me into a large bathroom, where four tubs stand in a row. She undresses me, runs warm water in the tub, and puts me in it.

She begins, "Ruth, I know this is the first time you have gone to school away from home. You may have many hard lessons to learn here, such as how to get along with other girls and when to cooperate with them as well as when to stand up for your own rights. Always remember, Ruth, that as a person, you have a responsibility to yourself as well as to others."

When I lie in bed in the dark ward that night, the day's events flash before my eyes—my first glimpse of NEIL, meeting Miss Knight, and listening to Miss Bartlett's strange words. Then I think of Mother, Dad, and Dave (too old, now, to be called Budge) at home. Tears come and slowly make their way down my cheeks. It's safe to cry in the dark, where no one sees me. I finally fall asleep.

Six o'clock Sunday morning comes too early. A nurse with an old face calls me.

"Ruth, it's time to get up. Breakfast will soon be here."

I sit up wearily, look around the ward, and remember where I am.

"Where's Miss Bartlett?" I ask.

"She's on afternoons. I'm Miss Watson, your morning nurse. Now let me help you with your shoes and socks and put you in your chair. We'll go to the bathroom and then wash our hands and face. Then we'll have breakfast."

We? I think. Is she going to the toilet and then going to have breakfast with me?

No, Miss Watson doesn't join me in these activities. She wheels me to the bathroom. After washing my face, Miss Watson takes me back to the ward, where a food cart awaits. She pushes me up to a round table and sets a tray before me.

I taste the watery orange juice and then the oatmeal. It is cold and lumpy. Ugh! I push it away. Lefty jerks. My spoon flies out of my hand and lands in the oatmeal. Milk spatters everywhere.

"Stop playing in your oatmeal, Ruth Webb," says Miss Watson sternly. "Eat it!"

"No, I'm not and I won't!" I shout, feeling hot all over.

"Don't say no to me, young lady! I'll make you."

Miss Watson seizes my jaw with one hand and squeezes my mouth open.

She pours the cold oatmeal down my throat with the other hand. I choke and spit it up. She pours it right back down. I spit it up again. This happens two, three, five times. We both become exhausted.

"Here, here! What's going on?" cries a familiar voice. It is Miss Bartlett. "I'm here to pick up my check and I hear this rumpus going on. What's it all about?"

"Ruth refuses to eat her oatmeal," glares Miss Watson.

"Don't you think Ruth is old enough to choose her own breakfast?" asks Miss Bartlett softly. "There's plenty of other food for her to eat, like dry cereal, boiled eggs, toast, and jelly."

"I don't believe in pampering children!" grumbles Miss Watson as she stalks away.

Miss Bartlett gets a cold wash cloth and wipes my tears away.

"Now, what will you have for breakfast?"

"Egg and toast with jelly, please," I whisper.

Miss Bartlett nods her head and quickly fetches a hot, gleaming white egg, some warm toast, and jelly. Then she smiles and pats my shoulder. "Ruth, I'm going now. Take care."

Glancing at Anne, Sally, and Mary, Miss Bartlett waves her hand and says, "I'll see you all at two o'clock."

"Wow, Ruth, do you have a friend!" Anne lets out a long breath.

"Yeah, Ruth, watch out for Watson!" cautions Mary. "She'll be laying for you."

It is peaceful—and boring—all morning. The girls' doctor has seen Sally, Anne, and Mary, and they are allowed to go out in the yard. He has yet to call me, so I am stuck on the ward for the morning. I open my new book, *The Swiss Family Robinson*, which Mother gave me when we left the Antlers.

All at once, I feel someone looking at me. I look up and see Miss Watson.

"Put that book down," she commands sternly. "I want to talk to you."

Placing her hands on her hips, she continues. "You work fast in making yourself a nurse's pet, don't you, Little Miss Ruthie?"

I get red and struggle for words and finally stammer, "M . . . M . . . Miss Bartlett is good to all of us. I'm not her pet."

"You just watch it, Ruth Webb. I don't want to fuss with Miss Bartlett over you again." Miss Watson shakes a warning finger in my face and stomps off noisily.

I am perplexed and miserable. Why is Miss Watson blaming me? I haven't asked Miss Bartlett for any favors.

This question tumbles over and over in my mind during the rest of the day. This is the first time I have ever been blamed for a deed I didn't do, and I don't know how to handle my indignant feelings. Thinking about the problem momentarily overshadows my homesickness and the wish to be near Mother, Dad, and Dave.

The next day is Labor Day, and Dr. White finally sees me. He is a jolly little man with a big smile.

I immediately demand of him, "When do I go to school?"

Dr. White picks up the class schedule. "School starts tomorrow. You are in Miss Knight's seventh grade. Your class meets from 9:00 to 10:30 every morning."

My heart sinks. Only one and a half hours of school a day. How can I learn anything in that time?

"Will I get physical therapy? I want to learn to walk!" I venture.

"Yes," Dr. White says. "Miss Carr, our therapist, has a full schedule right now, but she'll take you as soon as she can."

Seeing my face fall, Dr. White adds hastily, "It won't be long before Miss Carr has you walking."

I have no trouble getting up at six o'clock the next morning. I can hardly wait to join the other students in wheelchairs and bed cots as they wheel their way to the U-shaped brick school building.

Miss Knight greets me at the classroom door and assigns me a seat I can easily transfer to from my wheelchair. Miss Knight then introduces everybody. I tell the class I have come to NEIL to go to school and to learn to walk. At the time, I wonder why some of my classmates snicker at my remarks.

A month quickly passes. I am still at the Smyth Infirmary, and still not going to physical therapy. Although Miss Bartlett repeatedly warns me not to become dependent on her, I get very attached to her. We have long talks together and laugh a lot. I don't miss Mother, Dad, and Dave except after lights-out at night.

Then one afternoon Aunt Ethel pops in. After hugging me, she exclaims, "Ruthie, why aren't you in a cottage yet? I'll see about this!" And see about it, she does!

That very afternoon Aunt Ethel helps me move to C-4, an elbow-shaped, two-story cottage. When we enter the front door, we are in a large living room. Some older girls are huddled around a radio. Miss Brenda Berry, the head matron, greets me saying, "So you are Ruth Webb. We've been waiting for you. Come this way to your room."

With these few words, she leads us into the left wing of the cottage. Turning into the last room on the left side of the hall, Miss Berry points to the bed near the window. "This is your bed," she says. "You share the room with Betty Whitaker and Agnes Dobbs." Saying this, Miss Berry disappears.

I don't want Miss Bartlett to leave, and I cry when we say goodby. She promises to visit me. Her last words ring in my ears: "Remember to stand up for yourself."

Aunt Ethel hugs me and leaves with her.

A young matron in white enters the room. "I'm Miss Crawford," she says. "I'll help you unpack." She quickly puts my things away. Then she says, "Ruth, come with me and meet the living room girls." In the living room, she announces to the residents, "This is Ruth Webb, our new girl. Introduce yourselves to her."

"I'm Winnie Brant, president of C-4," says a heavyset girl, standing with crutches and long leg braces. "You're a spastic! Can you talk at all?" she asks scornfully.

Before I can answer, a girl in a high-backed wheelchair says, "My name's Roberta Elgin. You're the only spastic in the cottage. Most of us are polios."

One by one each of the ten living room girls tells me her name and disability and indicates disdain for "spastics."

The last one finally speaks. "I am Mary Paris. My polio only made my right foot smaller than my left one, so I just limp. You are in the seventh grade with me, aren't you?"

I nod and she continues. "I hear you're only twelve. You must be damn smart to be in the seventh grade. I'm nearly seventeen and I'm only in seventh this year."

"You should be downstairs with the playroom kids," growls Winnie. "But since you're in the seventh grade, I'll let you stay up here."

All this time I haven't said a word. I am afraid of Winnie and the living room girls. I edge over to the window and stay there until someone downstairs calls, "Supper!"

I look at the gray quartz ramp leading down to the basement. It's going to be hard to get back up this ramp, I think to myself. This flash of foresight proves correct. Were it not for our kindly janitor, Mr. Durham, we five wheelchair girls would never get back upstairs after meals. On his days off, we sometimes wait an hour or more before one of the matrons pushes us up the long, steep ramp. The basement floor is made of red bricks. We enter the dining room from the playroom, and Miss Crawford parks me at the end of a table.

Not many days pass before I realize that C-4 girls survive on a menu which is invariably the same for each day of every week. We always know what we are having for dinner and supper. Saturday is the worst dinner of all. The odor of cooking cabbage permeates the entire cottage all morning. The strong smell makes me ill, and I cannot eat (even to this day!) an "Irish" dinner of corned beef and boiled cabbage.

Almost all the living room girls except me are assigned household chores. I feel left out as I watch the others sweep and dust the hall and vacuum the living room. I am not a full member of the cottage because I have no job. The girls seem to look down on me because I don't share the work load.

After many months of feeling left out, I muster courage to ask Miss Berry if I can clean the ten wash basins in the basement rest room. She agrees to let me try. I am overjoyed and zealously scrub the sinks with sand soap every morning. The day even comes when Miss Berry scolds me for leaving a dirty basin. I am curiously proud. I am being yelled at just like any of the other girls.

I have a tough time getting used to the all-day-long scolding from our matrons, Miss B. Berry and Miss J. Berry. The living room girls call them the Bumble Bee and the Blue Jay.

In the living room, I learn much about campus boy-girl escapades. Gossip about clandestine meetings is gleefully passed from mouth to mouth, and happenings in secret rendezvous are magnified with each telling. I am thoroughly disgusted!

Most annoying are the soap operas which blare into the living room, one right after the other, every weekday afternoon. I get tired listening to the love crises that Stella Dallas and Old Ma Perkins get into. The girls never listen to the news or discuss politics, as Mother and Dad do at home.

After two days of nonstop melodramas, I retreat to my room. The first afternoon, I write letters on my dial typewriter. I am busily pounding the letters out on paper when Miss B. Berry sticks her head in the door.

"Ruth, you'll have to stop that now. This is my rest period. I can't sleep with that noise! Why don't you go out in the living room with the other girls?"

I stop typing, but I don't go to the living room. I stay in my room every afternoon and write letters by hand. Miss B. tells me not to seal them because Miss Smokestead, the girls' supervisor, reads them before sending them out. I wonder why we are not trusted to write uncensored letters.

As the days pass, I get more and more homesick. I miss everyone at home, but I miss Mother most of all. How I wish Miss Bartlett were here so I could talk to her. I feel so alone.

One day when I'm in my room, Miss Bartlett appears and scolds me for being sad. "Count your blessings, Ruth," she says. "You are in a new cottage. You could have been sent to the old ramshackle North Ward. Here in C-4, you have a chance for a decent life."

"B . . . b . . . but the girls don't like me!" I stammer.

"Have you tried to make friends with them?" she asks sternly.

"Y . . . y . . . yes," I answer.

"Then why are you in your room and not in the living room?"

"Because I like to read and write letters, and I can't do that in the living room. Besides, I don't like the stuff they listen to on the radio. You told me to make choices for myself."

Miss Bartlett puts her arm around my shoulders. "Yes, I told you to be responsible for yourself. But part of self-responsibility is making friends with the other girls. You'll have to assert yourself to find your own place in the group. Take that responsibility for yourself. No one can do the job for you. I'm counting on you to become a happy C-4 girl. Don't let me down!" Saying this, she kisses me and leaves. I never see her again, but I later recognize her words as utterances of the first of many spirit guides.

I do try to join the living room girls. Fitting in is always an uphill battle, and many times in my three years at NEIL, I become exhausted from the struggle. It never enters my mind to tell Mother and Dad about these problems. My surface excuse for this silence is that I don't want to worry Mother. Down deep, I don't want to

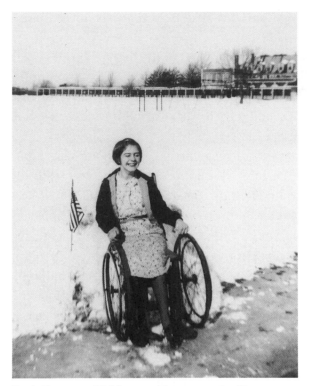

Ruth Cameron Webb, age thirteen, at the New England Institute for Learning, c. 1936

admit that Mother is right in not wanting me to go away from home.

Then I find a comforting retreat in the school's library, which is about fifteen feet from C-4's side door. Mrs. Price, the librarian, is a grandmotherly sort of person who at once takes me under her wing and encourages me to continue reading classical literature. The living room girls think I'm weird to read such books and tease me unmercifully. Nevertheless, I continue reading the classics. After all, Mother introduced me to these good books, and Mrs. Price is giving me the chance to continue to enjoy them.

As winter draws near and the weather gets colder, another problem plagues me. At the age of ten, a bad case of flu settled in my bladder, and ever since, cold temperatures have made me urinate with a very uncomfortable and inconvenient frequency.

Every morning the matrons open the ventilators in the roof to let in the chilly air. Because I am cold all day, I begin wetting my bed at night. When the heat is turned down to fifty degrees, I shiver in my bed under only two thin blankets. My urge to go is constant and painful.

The night nurse makes rounds only every two hours, so there is no one to help me to the bathroom. I try hard not to void but finally have to. I feel momentary relief, but the urge comes again and the miserable pattern is repeated over and over throughout the night. I finally fall asleep in the early morning, only to be awakened by the accusing cry, "Ruth Webb, you've wet your bed!"

That cry is soon echoed throughout C-4. The big girls laugh scornfully and tease me all through breakfast. "Now you have to have a rubber sheet on your bed. You think you're so smart, reading those dumb books. Shame on you!"

Sure enough, when Miss Crawford comes to make my bed, she brings a rubber mat and a draw sheet.

"When you learn not to wet your bed, we'll take these off," she says.

"I didn't wet my bed on purpose!" I exclaim. "I have a cold in my bladder."

"That's your story. I don't believe it." She taunts me, casting a knowing smile at the girls gathering at my door.

"Ruth Webb wet her bed. Ruth Webb wet her bed," chant the onlookers.

"I couldn't help it. I have a cold."

"Ruth Webb wet her bed," chant the girls again.

I begin to cry. My integrity as a person is threatened. For many days, I am ashamed to look the big girls in the eye.

No matter how hard I try to be accepted, problems with the big girls keep cropping up. There are bitter complaints from the other wheelchair users when I get two baths a week while they get only one. Jealous feelings against me reach raging force because Miss Bruner, a new matron, offers to walk me up and down the hall in the evening. When she realizes that her attention brings terrible wrath on me, this kind lady no longer walks me.

When Mother and Dave join Dad in Worcester and I return from weekend visits bringing apples, grapes, and giant Hershey bars (all of which I eat alone in the storeroom), the living room residents call me a pig. I am dimly conscious that Mother's goodies mean more than food to me; they symbolize that, in spite of my outcast role in the cottage, I am loved at home. The power of these treats is so strong that I even eat them after Thanksgiving dinner—and then throw up—much to the audible disgust of Miss Crawford.

My weekend trips increase jealous and scornful feelings toward me and revive my old habit of crying when waiting. Whenever Mother or Dad is fifteen minutes late in picking me up on Friday afternoons, I become panicky and start to cry. Severe chiding by my critics increases my anxiety and makes me cry harder.

At times I wonder if Grandpa's assurance that Jesus would always be with me can be true. If He really is my Guide, He isn't near me now.

I do have one girlfriend in C-4. My roommate, Betty, and I spend many afternoons in our room, chatting about this and that. We listen to each other's problems and remark on the doings of the matrons and the big girls. She has no trouble understanding my speech, as the others do. Betty is the person who saves me from feeling completely rejected in the cottage.

Sitting in a wheelchair all day does not improve my walking. Nine months pass before Miss Carr schedules me for therapy. Then I visit her three times a week. With Miss Carr right behind me, I soon again am taking twenty-five steps by myself.

My old bugaboo, space, continues to scare me and to retard my progress. Whenever I feel that Miss Carr is not near enough to catch me if I fall, my whole body tenses with fright. The cold sweat of fear rises in me. My right ankle turns and I stand, rooted to the floor, unable to move until Miss Carr puts a hand on my shoulder and says, "Relax, Ruth!" Miss Carr and I become great friends, and she tries hard to get me walking.

However, I never walk at NEIL. Mother claims that my nine months without walking practice prevented my further progress. She declares, "If you had been home, I would have made sure that you practiced daily, and you would have learned to walk."

The physical therapy sessions with Miss Carr make me an unwilling participant in frequent clinics for young doctors in Worcester. At these meetings, patients are paraded before thirty or more strange men in white coats while Dr. White comments upon the individual's condition.

Before "going onstage," I am completely undressed and clothed in a binder, gown, and robe. The latter two garments are hastily taken off when I am wheeled into the room. Icy chills go up my spine as I sit thus exposed for ten to fifteen minutes.

Dr. White at last acknowledges my presence by saying, "Here we have a spastic child with poor speech and involvement of all four extremities. We are teaching her to walk. Stand up, Ruth, and show them how you walk." He takes my hands and pulls me to my feet and walks me around the room. The doctors watch my naked body perform its awkward movements.

One particular clinic stands out in my memory. While I wait my turn, I watch my naked classmate Mildred, a tall lanky girl, badly deformed with arthritis, limp around the circle of doctors. Her face is a dull red with shame and embarrassment. This dehumanizing scene haunts me for many years.

Because the school laundry washes only two outfits a week for each student, I adopt the big girls' practice of washing my panties each night and hanging them on the bathroom's radiators to dry.

One day as I am washing my clothes, Miss B. appears in the doorway. "What are you doing, Ruth?" she asks.

"Washing my undies," I reply.

"You're supposed to wash clothes in the scrub sink, not in a wash

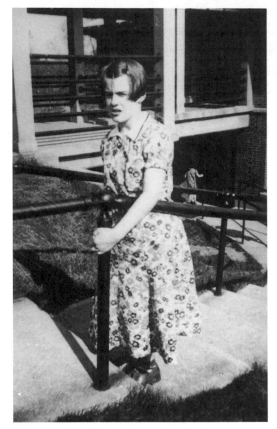

Ruth Cameron Webb, age fourteen, at the New England Institute for Learning, c. 1937

bowl," she says sternly. "Don't let me catch you washing in a bowl again."

I'll have to stand up to wash, I think.

The next day I'm standing at the sink when Miss B. again accosts me. "Ruth Webb, I told you not to wash your clothes in here."

"You said to wash in the scrub sink, not in the wash bowl," I protest.

"Humph! So I did. I didn't think you could stand." With these words, Miss B. leaves me forever alone to wash my duds.

The year wears on. I become quite despondent and read in my

room most afternoons. By now I am convinced that I never do any-thing right. The matrons don't seem to notice my distress. One day Dr. White catches me crying in my room and asks why, but he does nothing to help me.

I am happy only in class with Miss Knight. I excel in all subjects except spelling. Dad tells me not to worry. He is a poor speller too. So I let my spelling slip until I get a D. That mark makes me study my words, and I get an A on the next spelling test.

Miss Knight often gives us math homework. One day I find my interest problems in the living room wastebasket. Miss B. happens to be near and caustically remarks, "Oh, is that scribbling your homework? I thought one of the little kids was playing!"

I get red with anger but say nothing.

Sewing class is a good time. Miss Eton, a gentle-mannered lady, teaches me to weave on a hand loom. She threads the spindles in a prescribed pattern, and I push the shuttle back and forth through the strands of the warp. I make a green and white runner which becomes a knitting bag for Mother.

One day two tall ladies, friends of Aunt Ethel, visit me and invite me to spend the summer at Robin Hood's Barn, a camp for spastic children. I joyfully accept, since otherwise I would have to spend the entire summer at NEIL. Since Dad's retired from the Army in September 1935, he and Mother have been managing my grandma's summer inn, the Antlers.

When Dad drives me up to a little Vermont town in early July 1936 and leaves me at camp, I enter a fairy tale world. Gone are the matrons' day-long scoldings and the ceaseless criticisms from the big girls. Gone is the anxious fear that I will do something wrong.

At Robin Hood's Barn, each camper, as well as each counselor, lays aside his or her accustomed role and becomes one of Robin Hood's merry men. We even wear Lincoln green.

This ingenious idea to enable spastic children to experience life beyond their handicaps was developed by two special education teachers who called themselves Robin Hood and Little John.

Unknown to either of these ladies or to my parents and Aunt Ethel, living as Queen Eleanor, or "Queena," for eight weeks that summer restores my self-confidence.

I am Queen Eleanor not only in name. With my counselor, Maid Marian, in attendance, I have the power to choose what I want to do. Every day brings a new activity, a new experience. I finger paint, weave paper mats, and climb the jungle gym. I go on my first hay ride and stay awake until dawn on an all-night camp-out.

I even adapt the story of Cinderella to play format and then direct and act in the production. My thirteen years make me a bit old for some of these activities, but since I never have participated in them, they present delightful challenges.

How I dread the end of camp and my return to C-4. I console myself that I will be in the eighth grade, NEIL's senior class. I can never tell anybody in C-4 about Robin Hood's Barn. The living room girls would surely laugh in scorn at that imaginary world. Nonetheless, I feel stronger and more self-confident. I can now fight for my rights.

The eighth grade brings two hours of school every afternoon, weekly teas for NEIL staff, and monthly class meetings in the evening. Two mornings a week are spent in sewing class, and we attend a half-hour music class once a week. I spend most of this free time reading Shakespearean plays in my room or in the library.

We feel very important as we attend the first of our monthly class meetings held in the evening. This evening we elect officers, and I am chosen class historian. Miss Knight suggests that we adopt the Latin words *Per Aspera ad Astra* (Through Difficulty to the Stars) for our class motto.

Our weekly service project gives us girls experience and responsibility in serving tea to staff members. Each Friday afternoon, two girls dress in their Sunday best and take turns pouring tea from the big silver pot and dispensing cookies in the reception parlor of the administration building. Although I cannot pour tea or pass cookies, I preside as hostess once a month and greet our guests with a big smile.

One Friday as I go out the cottage front door, Winnie Brant approaches and asks accusingly, "Ruth, why are you going to Miss Knight's tea with dirty socks? You are supposed to be spic and span for these affairs!"

I protest, "I changed my socks after dinner. I can't help it if my legs go up in the air and rub my socks against the tires of my chair." I begin to cry.

"Oh hush, Crybaby! You'll never be anything but a spastic." Winnie puts her crutches under her arm and scornfully ambles in the front door of C-4.

When I get to the parlor in the administration building, I try to hide my dirty socks under the serving table.

The next never-to-be-forgotten event is a class trip to a circus animal training farm. After a three-hour ride through Massachusetts and New Hampshire, we arrive at the Circus Animal Farm. We eat a quick lunch and then walk through many buildings and outdoor enclosures. We see lions, tigers, elephants, monkeys, horses, and dogs, and we watch in awe as they perform their acts.

One event stands out from all the other dazzling sights I see that day. While we are waiting to board the bus for the homeward journey, Mr. Cabot, our guide, comes up to me and puts a little brown and black monkey in my lap. Its soft warm body snuggles against me.

"You may have the monkey if you want it. Her name is Sheba. She'll make you a nice pet." Mr. Cabot smiles.

I look longingly at the wee monkey and think, What would Miss B. say? I slowly shake my head and whisper, "No, thank-you!"

All the long bus ride home I wish I could have said yes.

The next morning we assemble on the schoolhouse lawn for the taking of our senior class picture. I am proudly wearing the white organdy dress that I basted together in sewing class. The picture of the class of 1937 still hangs in the schoolhouse hall at NEIL.

On the morning of graduation day, I learn in plain words what the big girls think of me. I am scrubbing the wash basins in the basement when I hear two big girls discussing the prestigious scholarship prize. "I know Ruth Webb is smart, but I think Helen Johns is smarter," says the first voice.

"Don't be too sure," rejoins her companion. "Didn't Ruth get the highest grade in the class on the final exam?"

"Only two points more than Helen. They won't give that prize to Ruth. Don't forget, she's a spastic," exclaims the first derisively.

Oh, I hope I show you! I think glumly.

Then a disturbing thought pops into my mind. What am I going to do after graduation? I try to push the idea away but it insists on returning. What will I do next year? I sure don't want to stay here another year. I want to go to high school.

Graduation night finally arrives. Our class president welcomes the guests, and we launch into our program of choral speaking. We recite Lincoln's Gettysburg Address, "Little Boy Blue" by Eugene Fields, and the thirteenth chapter of First Corinthians.

Next Miss Knight steps onstage to announce the winner of the scholarship prize. "This year we are indeed fortunate to have not only one but two excellent scholars in our graduating class. Both of these students have done such fine work that the trustees have decided to award a giant edition of Webster's Dictionary to each of these outstanding students, Helen Johns and Ruth Webb."

This is indeed a triumphant moment. I look toward the C-4 girls. They are cheering madly—I hope for both Helen and me.

Mother and Dad promise to find a high school for me if I stay at NEIL one more year while Dad finishes his master's degree in education at Harvard University. Mother is supplementing the family's income by selling *My Bookhouse for Children*, a set of twelve volumes containing the world's great classical literature, graded for children from infancy through high school.

I reluctantly agree to take typing and English literature with Miss Knight, but I am bored and unhappy that grad year at NEIL. I yearn for the day I will go home for good with Mother, Dad, and David. Time passes slowly in spite of my forays into *Beowulf* and Robert Browning.

One night I dream Aunt Ethel will take me home to my parents in the morning. Lo and behold, my dream comes true the very next day. At 11:30 A.M., I am in my room reading Milton's *Paradise Lost*. The phone rings and I hear Miss B. call out in her raucous voice, "Ruth Webb going home for good!" It is the cry I have yearned to hear for three long, weary years.

This day I leave C-4 and my minority role forever. The first painful steps of my journey, taken with shame and rejection, are over. But they leave shadows. There are many nights in which the Berry sisters and the big girls haunt my dreams. The three years in which "I never do anything right" bequeath a lasting impression of inferiority.

Now, however, I am happy. It is September 1939, and I am going home to Swarthmore, Pennsylvania, with Mother, Dad, and Dave. Best of all, I am going to high school. I'm sure of it!

3

Wending My Way through Latin and Other Lessons

After the boring and unproductive grad year at NEIL, I am frantic to go to high school—anywhere!

While searching for a suitable high school, Mother hears about the Citizens' Rehabilitation Institute in Maryland. This pioneer school offers physical and occupational therapy *and* a high school education to students with cerebral palsy.

Dr. Winthrop Phelps, a tall slim man with a bald head and smiling blue eyes, greets us as we mount white marble steps and enter the end door of one of Baltimore's famous block houses. He ushers us into his office–examining room, and when we are seated, he takes my complete medical history and then gives me an orthopedic examination. He speaks softly to me in a shy confidential way, and I feel comfortable as he moves my limbs this way and that.

When the exam is over and I am dressed again, Dr. Phelps sits in a chair next to me and says, "Ruth, I think we can get you walking—and you can go to high school at my school, which we call CRI."

I look at Mother and Dad. They are beaming. Then Mother asks anxiously, "What is the tuition?"

"Four hundred a month," replies Dr. Phelps. "This covers room, board, housemother care, and schooling, as well as physical, occupational, and speech therapy. A full training schedule."

Mother says to Dad, "Billy, I can earn the money by selling more sets of *My Bookhouse*. I know I can!" And so I go to CRI in February 1939, while Mother sells books to keep me there.

My dream of attending high school is finally fulfilled. I take to my long-sought curriculum as a duck to water. I fall in love with Miss Hart, my English, French, and Latin teacher, and young Mr. Bruce, who teaches algebra and biology, fascinates me.

I am thrilled when I translate my first words in Latin, *Sicilia est una insula*, to mean "Sicily is an island."

Both Miss Hart and Mr. Bruce give homework to me and the other high school students. Every weeknight we have study hall in Miss Hart's room, and I enjoy greatly translating a short story in Latin, memorizing French irregular verbs, reading biology, and solving algebra equations.

Mr. Polling, administrator of CRI, often monitors our evening study hall. He is always a kind friend and wise counselor, and in my three years at CRI, I become very fond of him.

In addition to my cherished high school program, I also start to work on learning to walk. Fran Presser, a slim, dark-haired girl in her twenties, is my first physical therapist. When she learns of my burning desire to walk, she promises to do all she can to put me on my feet.

Fran defines my disability in new ways and calls me a person *with* cerebral palsy, not a cerebral-palsied person. She says I have athetosis, Dr. Phelps's term for my involuntary movements. Fran

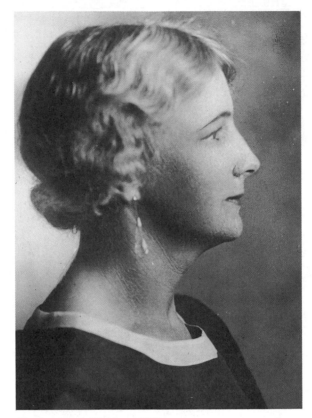

Mother Ruth Webb, c. 1939

explains that my arms flap out at my sides when I try to raise them above my head because the message centers in my brain are jumbled.

I am a "mixed case" because I have athetoid movements with tension in all four limbs and spasticity in my right ankle and heel cord. Under physical and psychological stress, such as walking in a large, open space or anticipating an important exam, the spastic muscles draw my heel up till I'm standing on my toes. Then the spastic ankle kicks in and pulls my foot over on its outside. My foot hurts with a hot band of tension wrapping around my ankle and spreading up my leg.

Fran's remedy for this muscular impasse is to teach me voluntary relaxation. Fran first massages my trunk and limbs. She then asks me to tense and relax each muscle group in my body.

Before beginning walking practice with me, she teaches me to fall without hurting myself. She stands me on a thick mattress and tells me to pretend I'm a rag doll and to fall limply on the soft mattress. When I realize that mattress falls don't hurt, I relax and enjoy the experience.

When I take steps by myself, Fran is always close behind me. The instant she moves an inch or two away from me, I tense with shivers of fear, my right ankle turns, and I start to fall. Of course, Fran always catches me, but still I tremble with fear when I stand alone in "empty" space, with nothing around me.

Constant practice in taking steps on my own leads to the day I walk forty-five steps down the hall leading to my classroom. Space in this narrow passageway is not scary because the walls are close together and the ceiling is low. On the other hand, the fifty-foot reception hall frightens me terribly. Built to be used as a ballroom, it measures fifty by one hundred feet, and its only furniture consists of four yellow velveteen couches on each side of the room. Its dark vaulted ceiling adds to my feeling of being out in space, and I hesitate to stand in it.

One day Fran decides I should go solo in this immense hall. "Ruth, I'm going to stand here by the couch and you're going to walk across the reception room without me behind you," she announces decisively. "If you fall, I'll catch you. But you can walk to me all by yourself. I know you can."

I never forget the agonizing moments of that first twenty-five-foot walk alone. Fear makes me sweat with cold chills. How I struggle to reach Fran on the far side of the hall. I take two steps, then look at the couch on the other side of the room. My right leg tenses and my foot becomes rooted to the floor. I look down quickly. The troublesome ankle turns completely over and cramps terribly. My heart thumps with fear and I ache all over.

"Ruth, relax that ankle. Let it straighten up," Fran coaches.

I try to make the tightness release my ankle. I stand looking at the floor, afraid to look at the empty space around me. Five agonizing moments tick slowly by. Fran continues to urge me to relax my foot and to come to her. Finally my ankle straightens a bit and I take four slow steps. My heel rises again and turns on its side.

"Relax, Ruth!" warns Fran. "Head up. Look at me."

Some more minutes pass. My foot relaxes again. I raise my head and look at Fran. She spreads her arms wide. With a choking sob, I take the three remaining steps and fall into her arms. She hugs me tightly while tears stream down both our faces.

So I walk at age seventeen. It is truly an overwhelming moment for both Fran and me. Although fear continues to haunt my steps in large spaces, I now know I can fight it and win.

Time passes, and one day Fran brings me a tripod walker, made of one-inch pipe. Joining the three legs is a wooden handle, just large enough for my left hand. I affectionately call it the crab, and it gives me the support and confidence I need to walk alone in space.

When I am finally walking with the crab, getting up from the floor after a tumble becomes a crucial problem. One morning Fran says, "Ruth, I think I've worked out your getting-up movements. Stand on your knees and put your weight on your left leg. Then straighten it and pull up on the crab. There, now you've risen from the floor all by yourself."

Fran is not the only one to teach me important lessons. Ellie Yates of the Occupational Therapy Department helps me gain daily living skills. Tying my shoes is the first problem she tackles. Ellie solves it by making my shoelaces uneven and teaching me to tie a one-bow knot.

Ellie introduces me to the electric typewriter. At first, I make many errors because of the fast action of the keys. When I learn to use a quicker touch, I type a double-spaced page in an hour with only one error. A new way to communicate opens for me. I think that perhaps this new typewriter will help me go to college.

Mrs. Darwin, my first housemother, is also an important person in my life. It is she who suggests I try walking alone in the two-foot space between beds in our dormitory. To my great delight, the closeness of the beds dissipates my fear of space, and I have no trouble walking in the narrow passageway.

My roommate, Cory, has grown up in a school for retarded children and feels rejected by her father. Her mother cares about her, but her dad seems reluctant to pay for her tuition at CRI. He grudgingly agrees to fund Cory's training only for six months. If she doesn't learn to walk in that time, he will put her in a mental institution.

During the next six months, I watch Cory anxiously as she struggles in vain to learn to walk. Cory has trouble keeping her balance between steps. As she walks, she goes faster and faster until her feet fly out from under her and she falls in a heap.

One day when we are alone, Cory voices her fear. "Ruth, I'm so afraid if I don't walk soon, my father will take me out of CRI and put me in an institution and leave me there forever." She begins to cry. "Why can't I learn to walk like you? I get mad when I see you walk."

"Your mother won't let you be put in an institution," I exclaim. Watching her panic grow, I gain a better appreciation of my own parents. Mother is selling books door to door to keep me in school and I know Dad will give up everything to see me walk.

Because of her mother's pleading, Cory remains in school for two years. After her mother dies of cancer, Cory's dreaded nightmare comes true. Placed in a "Home for Incurables," she begins to act out her deep anger with violent rages. Unable to cope with such behavior, the Home dismisses her, and she lands in a state mental institution. Cory dies there after three years, angry and lonely.

One member of our high school group, Rollo Balk, seems to like me a lot. He is a good student, and we often stay after study hall to talk. Our companionship blossoms into a comfortable friendship. We see politics and current events in the same way, and we are both concerned about preparing for and getting a job.

One afternoon in Miss Hart's room, we high schoolers have a

meeting and agree to form a club "to entertain and educate its members." I suggest we call ourselves "The Hi Steppers" as a reminder of our ambitious plans for the future. This idea meets with general approval, and we proceed to elect officers. Rollo is chosen president and Dee, my roommate, is elected vice-president. I am secretary-treasurer. Miss Hart agrees to be club advisor.

We meet once a month on Monday nights. A never-to-be-forgotten occasion is the evening Rollo and I re-enact the balcony scene from Shakespeare's *Romeo and Juliet*. Miss Hart gives us a two-page script in American-Italian dialect to which we add our cerebral-palsied speech. The play takes place in the physical therapy room. The top landing of the practice stairs makes a realistic balcony for me as Juliet.

The scene opens as the heroine just barely manages to gasp out between giggles: "Romeo, Romeo, where in the heck did you get to, Romeo?"

The very select audience (Miss Hart and the other three Hi Steppers) roars with laughter as Romeo replies, "I'm right under you, mia lovey. Throw me a kissy. Please!"

"You can't catch my kissies. They bounce!" declares Juliet. "Come to me, mio lovey. I yearn to hug you."

"What?" exclaims the astonished Rollo, forgetting he is Romeo.

Then clomp, clomp. His heavy shoes ascend the seven steps to Juliet's landing. He spreads his long gangling arms to enclose her, thereby letting go of the side railings. The next moment Romeo falls to his knees on the step immediately below the landing. Shaken but with great stage presence, Romeo cries desperately, "Sweet Juliet, see how your Romeo falls for you. Gimme a kissy. Please!"

Amid the great burst of laughing and clapping, Romeo reaches up, clasps Juliet's neck, and plants a loud juicy kissy on her nose!

"I will do the kissing, mio Romeo!" declares the actress.

Then the furiously blushing Juliet shoves Romeo away with such angry force that he slides down the seven steps on his knees.

When he reaches the floor, Romeo rises up on his knees. He mutters, "Sweet Juliet, just one sweet bouncy kissy from you sure makes me fall!"

This moment is enshrined forever in the collective memory of the Hi Steppers.

Not long after this dramatic moment, one evening after study hall, Rollo hands me an obscene note. Frightened by its implication, I give the note to Mr. Polling. I am bewildered. Can it be that Rollo wants to have sex with me? Why? I'm not even sure what having sex involves. Mother has always refused to discuss the matter with me.

Thereafter, Rollo is closely guarded and is finally dismissed from CRI. He writes me for many years and even invites me to collaborate with him on my autobiography. I never agree to his repeated requests.

One of the enterprises spawned by the Hi Steppers is a monthly paper dubbed the *Institute Informer*. For most of the two years of the *Informer's* existence, we meet on Sunday afternoons to plot the next issue and to give writing assignments. As editor, I write the feature stories and organize the makeup of the eight-page, two-column paper. The *Informer* reports on current events and excursions and advertises essay and carryover contests.

The latter event is an annual attempt to get students to practice skills they are learning in physical therapy. Staff members record the times they see students practicing carryover skills. Each week the student receiving the most check marks attends a restaurant dinner with Mr. Polling.

One year I win this contest by keeping my head up when I walk. It is a great thrill to eat in a real restaurant and to choose my dinner from twelve entrées. While we eat, Mr. Polling tells funny stories and ignores my silence. I cannot talk while eating.

After my last bite of lemon pie is down, Mr. Polling lights his dark walnut pipe. Exhaling a few fragrant puffs, he looks straight into my eyes and asks, "Ruth, what are you going to do after high school?"

"I'm going to college," I quickly reply.

"And then what will you do?" queries Mr. Polling.

"Er . . . I want to be a teacher. I'm going to teach c.p. kids."

"How will you handle kids in wheelchairs and run after those who walk?"

"Don't teachers have aides?" I ask dubiously.

"Not every teacher is that lucky. Beginning teachers almost never have aides."

"Then I can't be a teacher?" I ask, drawing a painful breath.

"I didn't say that," Mr. Polling protests. "I'm just trying to make you think of some of the problems you will face in getting and keeping a job."

"But if I go to college, I'm sure to get a job, aren't I?" I blurt out.

Mr. Polling sighs. "Ruth," he says softly, "why do you want a job? Why not stay home and—"

"And read? I've been told that before!" I fairly shout. "No, I'm going to help others. I want my life to count for something."

"Hold on, Ruth! I'm just warning you not to try to reach unrealistic goals. You must select your vocational goals carefully to maximize your assets and minimize your limitations."

"But how will I know what goals are unrealistic before I try to reach them?" I demand.

Mr. Polling chuckles. "Good thinking, Ruth! Just remember to use your good brain when you plot your life's course between the peaks of lofty ambition and the rocks of hard knocks."

All the way back to CRI, I hear Mr. Polling's words—"Maximize your assets and minimize your limitations"—and wonder what they mean.

What are my assets? Do I have any? I can write a little, but can I make a living by writing? Do I want to write all the time? No, I want to help people.

And my limitations? Will my cerebral palsy stand in the way of my becoming a real professional? Will people understand my speech? How will I get to work if I can't drive a car?

Thoughts concerning my future focus my attention on God. Why did He create me? Why am I handicapped? Does God have a purpose for my life? These questions whirl in my brain all day long and keep me awake far into the night.

Finally I get enough courage to tell Mr. Polling about my agonizing questions. He at once asks the Methodist minister in the village to call on me. I prepare for his visit by writing down my questions.

The appointed hour comes at last. I meet the Rev. Jefferson in the front parlor. He is a portly, middle-aged gentleman with twinkling blue eyes and a hearty laugh.

He shakes my hand, sits down, and begins at once. "I understand you have some hard questions for me, Ruth. Let's have them."

I hand him my list. "Can you read my writing, Sir?" I ask timidly.

"Yes, indeed! Hmmm, you ask some very crucial questions. Let me deal with them one by one."

He reads, "Why did God create me?"

He looks at me tenderly. "Dear Ruth, the Lord created human beings to be His companions. He loves us and wants us to return His love. He created you to love Him."

"God needs love!" I exclaim. "I thought only we humans need love from God—not the other way around!"

Mr. Jefferson declares, "In any relationship, love must be both given and received. God gives you the ability to return the love He gives to you, if you so wish."

"If God loves me, then why did He let me be handicapped? I'd be easier to love if I could walk and talk like other kids."

"Dear Ruth, when the Lord first created us, He laid down certain rules for human life which, when broken, bring sorry consequences. Because you were injured at birth, you can't walk or talk the way other folks do. But the Lord gave you a brain that can overcome the effects of the accident at birth."

"But does God have a purpose for *me*?" I ask.

He hesitates a moment, then begins again. "Yes, dear Ruth, God has a plan for each of us. Whatever the plan for you, you may be sure it includes relating to Him day by day."

"How do I relate to Him day by day?" I ask.

"Do you know Jesus Christ as your Lord?" the Rev. Jefferson queries softly. "Do you ever speak with Him?"

"Grandpa Webb told me about Jesus long ago," I answer. "I know He is my Lord, but I don't know that He talks to me."

"Dear Ruth, Jesus always listens when we call to Him. I don't mean that He completely removes our difficulties from us. Instead, Jesus helps us overcome problems as they occur, but we must want Him to be our Guide."

"How do I ask Jesus to be my Guide?" I whisper.

"Do you want me to pray that He will come into your heart and forevermore be your Guide?" asks the fatherly minister.

I nod, as tears run down my cheeks.

The Rev. Jefferson puts his hand on my head and prays. "Oh Lord, come and abide in your daughter, Ruth. Lord, she desires to be led by You. I pray Ruth will always call on You for guidance and that your Holy Spirit will ever help her through life's trials. Amen."

I have a sudden idea. "Rev. Jefferson, would I be nearer to Jesus if I join your church?"

His eyes twinkle again. "No, Dear, you are as near to Jesus now as you'll ever be. But I'd love for you to join our little church in Pikesville. Have you ever been baptized?"

"No," I answer.

"Then I'll arrange for you to be baptized and to join our church two weeks from next Sunday. I'll see you again before that to go over any questions you may have." Rev. Jefferson shakes hands and leaves.

And so it is that on a bright Sunday in April 1939 a seventeen-year-old girl in a pink suit and broad-brimmed hat is baptized and joins the little white frame Methodist church in Pikesville, Maryland. Mother and Dad come to witness the occasion.

As the water is sprinkled on my head and I repeat the vows of church membership, a calm, steady peace oozes up from the pit of my stomach and floods my chest with bubbling joy. At that moment, I know Jesus is with me.

Seeing my joy, Mother smiles with delight. Dad beams and proudly thumps me on my shoulder. "Pilikia, you're going to make it!" he whispers in my ear.

With the beginning of my last year in high school, I begin to wonder if I will get to go to college. My grade average is B+, high enough for acceptance by most colleges. But when the admissions officers look at my application and see the words *cerebral palsy*, they reject my application without ever seeing me. After five such refusals from colleges whose names are long forgotten, my spirits sink to suboceanic depths. I forget about calling on Jesus for help. I feel my life will unquestionably end if I don't go to college.

Finally, Dad calls me to say that he has found a college for me. He says excitedly, "Pilikia, Sanders College for Women in Riverside, Pennsylvania, has agreed to accept you on a trial basis."

"Will there be someone to help me?" I ask doubtfully.

"The dean of women has asked a student to room with you and help you. We will pay her tuition for the semester. Everything is all set for the beginning of a great college career for you."

Two weeks remain before I enter Sanders College. Hawkie, my housemother, hustles to pack my belongings. Fran gives me extra walking time in Physical Therapy to give my right leg practice in stepping forward. In Occupational Therapy, Ellie has me copy endless paragraphs on the electric typewriter to raise my speed and accuracy to the highest possible level. Mr. Foss, our teacher, reviews English and French grammar to prepare me for the all-important placement tests at college. Everybody is very excited that a CRI student is really going to college.

I float in a dreamy haze. It is Mr. Polling who brings me down to earth. The evening before I leave CRI, he takes me into the front parlor for a final chat.

"Ruth," he begins, looking earnestly at me. "You are a good student. We're proud of you and the fact that you've been accepted by a first-rate college. However, I feel that it is my job to warn you that things may not work out the way you plan."

"But Dad tells me everything is arranged. The college has accepted me and I have a roommate to help me. What can go wrong?"

"Lots of things, Ruth," Mr. Polling shakes his head. "You and your roommate may not get along. Your class schedule may be too physically tiring for you. You may not be able to complete written assignments on time. All I'm saying is this: Don't be too disappointed if this try at college doesn't work out. You can always return to CRI."

Come back to CRI? I wince at the thought. No, I won't be back. I'm going to college!

The great day comes on September 15, 1941. Dad drives me to the little town of Riverside. We turn in to the college grounds and park in front of a massive four-story structure. Dad walks me slowly along the twenty-five-foot gravel path. I am breathing hard, my palms are sweaty, and my right ankle tenses and turns over.

Just before we reach the door, Dad whispers in my ear. "Relax, Pilikia. Remember, not everyone is accepted as a freshman by Sanders College—and you are!"

Dad opens the big red door and we walk into a huge lounge. Dad seats me in the only straight chair available. The ceiling is very high and the room so wide and long. Its vastness summons my old fear of space and makes me tremble within. I keep my eyes on Dad and dare not look up toward the ceiling.

As Dad approaches a nearby office, the door swings open and a tall, gray-haired lady greets him. "You must be Mr. Webb and Miss Webb. I am Dean Harding, and I will show you your room and introduce you to your roommate, Rebecca Cooper."

Saying this, Dean Harding leads the way to a tiny elevator. "Your room and classes are all on the second floor. The only steps you will have are the three up into the dining room." This remark makes me a little uneasy, but I say nothing.

When the door opens, we follow Dean Harding to the second door beyond the elevator. The open door reveals a large room with a bay window. Two beds sit beside their respective desks and bookcases. It is indeed the college room of my dreams.

Just then, a girl with straight brown hair and hazel eyes walks in. She wears a big smile as she opens both arms to hug me.

"Ruth Webb, this is your roommate, Rebecca Cooper. She is a junior this year in the Education Department," declares Dean Harding enthusiastically. "You two are going to be great friends." She adds, "Mr. Webb and I are going to leave now. You girls need to get to know each other."

When the door closes, Rebecca turns to me and queries, "How do you get around? Do you walk at all?"

"I walk with help. Let me show you. Put your hand under my left arm and take my wrist. Then we can walk side by side."

Becky jumps up, grabs my wrist, pulls me to my feet, and starts to walk rapidly across the room. Immediately my body tenses and my right ankle turns over. I become breathless and therefore speechless. I lean perilously toward the right and my right foot is glued to the floor. Becky pulls on my left arm to straighten me up, and we both almost fall. She drags me at an agonizing speed toward my desk chair on the other side of the room.

I finally stammer, "B . . . B . . . Becky, don't go so fast! I have to relax."

Becky finally stops two feet from the desk. She pulls the chair up to me and sits me in it with a loud thump.

Sighing, she says, "Ruth, I don't think I can be your roommate. I can't help you walk. I'm so sorry." She turns away from me and starts to cry.

"Becky, you *can* help me walk! I'll show you how. You just have to wait between each step till I get my balance."

"But you lean too much on me," Becky breaks in. "I can't hold you up!"

"Give me time to relax and get my balance," I plead. "I can even walk alone if you don't hurry me."

"There are a lot of steps in these old buildings, including the ones to the dining room. They're rounded and made of tile. I'm not sure I can manage you up and down those steps."

"Please try. I want to stay here and go to college so bad."

"Well, this is Friday. I'll work with you till Sunday and try to learn how to help you walk. If not, well . . ."

Becky pauses and abruptly changes the subject. "Tomorrow morning you have a placement test in English at nine o'clock and one in French at ten o'clock. Let's see how we do about getting you to the classroom in Honegger Hall. Although our buildings are all connected, the Language Department is almost a block away. The trip will give us plenty of time to practice walking together."

Becky and I spend the rest of the afternoon unpacking and putting clothes in closets and drawers. While doing this, we chat, and by dinnertime we are fast friends. She now has little trouble understanding my speech, and we walk side by side around the room a dozen times. As she learns to wait for me to shift my balance between steps, we gain confidence in each other and my right ankle relaxes.

Becky and I walk to the dining room and ascend the three rounded marble steps without incident. We sit at a table set for nine with a white linen cloth and red napkins.

Young waitresses appear, bearing huge platters heaped high with golden fried chicken. I groan inwardly as I realize this is too formal a situation to pick the chicken up in Lefty's fingers. There are lovely green peas. My heart sinks. I can't possibly eat them with a fork! I look imploringly at Becky.

She smiles and says, "Ruth, may I cut your chicken?"

I smile and murmur, "Thank you."

The dinner proceeds without incident. I capture all my peas in the mashed potatoes and transport them successfully to my mouth. My fork has no trouble spearing the bite-size pieces of chicken. After dinner Becky asks a friend to help us down the three tile steps, and we walk slowly toward our room. I am very relaxed and confident, and Righty's ankle doesn't turn over once.

Becky and I spend the evening learning about each other. She likes dogs and cats and so do I. We both enjoy classical music and historical novels about women. Becky believes there is a God but is not sure where Jesus fits in. I *know* Jesus is God's son and my guide. We chat long after we are in bed. At last we go to sleep. I am happy. I have a new friend.

In the still dark morning while we are dressing, Becky says off-handedly, "Ruth, would you like me to bring your breakfast to the room? It would save time and be much easier for both of us."

I have no choice and agree, feeling very uneasy. So Becky goes to the kitchen and returns with boiled eggs and bacon, toast, and or-ange juice for both of us.

As we hurriedly eat, my roommate explains the purpose of the placement tests. "Entering students are tested for placement in lan-guage courses to see if they are ready for beginning, intermediate, or advanced language courses."

After a thirty-minute walk, we arrive at the Language Depart-ment. My right ankle hurts from tension but turns over only once. I'm breathing hard, and my stomach cramps with excitement.

When I am seated, the instructor hands me a printed test booklet and says, "Welcome to Sanders College English Placement Test. You have an hour and a half to complete this exam."

I have never taken a timed test before, and I get very tense. I grip my pencil hard and start on the vocabulary section. All items are multiple choice, and I manage to finish them within the allotted time.

The test is over, and the girls quickly file out of the room. As I wait for Becky, I see the teacher looking at my test. She walks over to me and whispers, "Congratulations, Miss Webb! You made an almost perfect score on the vocabulary section."

I almost burst with pride as I walk with Becky to the classroom where the French placement test is about to begin. After another successful experience with a timed test, Becky and I go to the din-ing room for lunch.

When lunch is over, we try to walk down the three tile steps without extra help. We almost succeed, but my right heel catches on the lowest tile step as we descend. I lurch forward and fall on my knees, dragging Becky down with me. A crowd of girls immediately gathers amid a noisy buzz. Becky and I are quickly raised to our feet by numerous hands. I am unhurt and start giggling. Becky isn't hurt either, and she joins me in giggling all the way back to our room.

Shortly after our return to our room, Dean Harding knocks at the door and says curtly, "Rebecca, I want to see you for a few minutes. Please come with me."

I wonder what is up, and the lump in my throat assumes golf-ball size before Becky comes back. She enters abruptly and slams the door and exclaims, "Harding, that old bag! She won't listen to me."

"W . . . w . . . what's the matter?" I stammer.

Becky gasps, "Oh, Dean Harding thinks you're too handicapped to go to college—this college anyway! She says you're too heavy for me to lug around. I tried to tell her I can manage you just fine, but she wouldn't listen. She heard about our fall in the dining room and decided you can't stay at Sanders." Becky breaks into tears. Sitting on my bed and hugging each other tightly, we both cry for what seems a long time.

Then Becky wipes her eyes and says, "Ruth, we have to pack your things. Dean Harding called your dad, and he will be here around four o'clock. We still have two hours to be together. Tell me all you can about what it's like to have cerebral palsy. I need to know if I'm going to be a special ed teacher."

Although I am totally without feeling, I do my best to comply with Becky's request. Two hours pass quickly. Becky is genuinely interested in how it feels to be handicapped, how I learn, how I deal with negative attitudes like the one Dean Harding is showing. We are discussing my three-legged cane when Dad walks in.

He hugs me and whispers, "You gave it your best shot, Pilikia. Don't worry, you'll have another chance to go to college. Remember Mommy's old slogan, and try, try again."

And then he adds, "I've just talked with Dean Harding. She's sorry things didn't work out. She says you made top scores on your

French and English tests, but taking care of you is just too much for Becky. She's also afraid of your falling in these old buildings. She doesn't want to upset you by saying good-by and asks me to tell you she admires you greatly."

"Humph! I bet!" I snort.

I give my college-room-for-a-night one last look and slowly walk out the door. Outside I look up at the second-floor windows and catch a glimpse of Becky waving. My college career is over.

At home there is nothing to do but feed the fires of indignation and anger kindled by my unjust expulsion from Sanders College. If only Dean Harding had let me stay just one week and attend classes. If only the dining room had had no steps. If only Becky had been larger and stronger. If only I could walk better. If only . . . if only.

Small flames of wrath, ignited and fed over the years by put-downs, both real and imagined, now gather into a huge conflagra-tion of resentment and perform a searing dance in my chest. Nega-tive questions overwhelm me again and again. Why do I live? If no college will train me, I can't be a teacher. I can't help c.p. kids. In fact, I can't help anyone. My life is a failure.

At home once more, I read. I can't write or even listen to my favorite record of "Swan Lake." Anger envelopes and suffocates me. I am paralyzed, unable to think or move. Even Dave cannot joke me out of this painful state.

It is Mother who rescues me from my self-inflicted wounds. One morning she walks into my room and says briskly, "Ruthie, it's time for you to shed your mourning cloak. Get out of this room and get on with your life. Just because one college rejects you is no reason to give up entirely. Come downstairs and into the kitchen with me. Your dad and I have an idea for you."

When he sees me, Dad gets up and pulls out a chair for me, say-ing, "Ruthie, how would you like to go back to CRI while Mother and I look for another college for you?"

Go back to CRI? After I left with such high hopes? Admit to Mr.

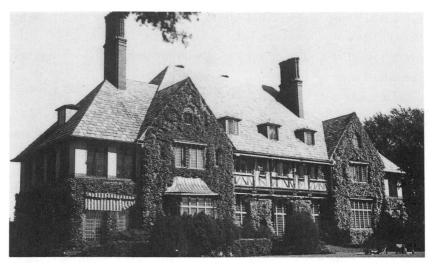

Citizens' Rehabilitation Institute, Baltimore, Maryland

Polling that his words, "Things may not work out," came to pass? Never!

"What will I do there?" I ask, looking at Dad.

"Continue physical and occupational therapy and take a college correspondence course. The Home Study Department of the University of Chicago offers courses in many areas. Let's send for a catalog and see what courses interest you," Dad answers.

The catalog comes in a few days. Dad and I leaf through it, and I select a course entitled "Introduction to Social Science." I agree to go back to CRI, but only until Dad finds another college. So, after three and a half months at home, I return to the site of my high school days with great sadness in January 1942.

Contrary to my expectations, Mr. Polling greets me warmly and doesn't mention my college "failure." He announces a big change in my room assignment by saying, "Ruth, you are so self-sufficient, you no longer need a housemother. You are going to live in the classroom wing with two other young ladies."

At first, I wander around CRI in a fog. One hazy day blends into the next. I half-heartedly try to improve my walking in Physical

Therapy and to increase my typing speed in Occupational Therapy. I read the textbook and receive A's and B's on the long and wearisome papers I write for my social science course, but nothing interests me.

I never smile or laugh. I cry often without apparent reason. I neglect my grooming. With no housemother to check up on me, my socks often don't match my dress—or indeed each other. My hair is not combed and my shoes are not polished. My clothes go unmended and I wear them that way. I just no longer care about ANYTHING!

One day I go to the Occupational Therapy shop, sit down before the typewriter, and weep. I feel so low, so sick, so desperate. Ellie takes one look at me, leaves for a moment, and returns with a wheelchair. "Ruth, we're going to have a talk!" she announces firmly.

In the empty office, we sit facing each other. Ellie's mouth is sternly set as she begins. "Ruth Webb," she says, "what is the matter with you? You used to be the best-dressed girl in school. Now look at you. Your blouse is missing at least two buttons and your skirt belt is twisted three or four times."

I hang my head and stammer. "I . . . I don't have anyone to fix my clothes!"

Ellie sniffs. "Have you asked anyone to fix your clothes?"

"I have no housemother."

"Umm, that is easy to remedy. I'll ask Mr. Polling to find someone to help you. Now what about your long face and ever-present tears? You know, Ruth, you have a responsibility to the other students to smile and be cheerful even though you're aching on the inside. You are a born leader. Everybody—staff and students—looks up to you. Don't let us and yourself down because you've had a little setback in your plans. Screw up your courage. Try again!" At this point, my mind echoes again with Mother's oft-repeated words, "Try, try again!"

Shame over my behavior and thankfulness for Ellie's caring words make me shed a few more tears. I finally stop crying. Ellie ends the meeting by giving me a big hug as she whispers, "Ruth, I *know* you're going to do great things!" Her words are remembered as a signpost marking the first time I acknowledged and gave thanks for the intervention of a spirit guide.

After that, things improve immensely. Sarah, my roommate, mends my clothes, and I no longer wear torn blouses or unmated socks. I make efforts to rise from my despondency, to keep myself clean and neat, to improve my typing and walking, and to earn an A in my correspondence course (I got a B+). I come out of myself and once more edit the *Institute Informer.*

And I am everlastingly grateful to Ellie, who leads me gently but resolutely out of my high school doldrums.

4

The Path through Two Colleges

"Come now, are you going to let me finish my twenty-five laps in the pool or do I have to stop and take you back to the room?" the husky girl demands threateningly.

September 1943 brings a trial acceptance by Angel College in Scranton, Pennsylvania. I am now twenty years old. In return for tuition, Penny Davenport has agreed to help me in my second attempt to attend college.

She and I are poolside in Angel College's new gym. I am fast learning that Penny is devoted to sports and not at all concerned about me. "I can't take care of you if you don't let me practice swimming. Now, are you going to be sick again or are you going to let me swim?" Penny shakes her finger at me.

The pool room seems tremendously large and has a very high

ceiling. It frightens me and makes me sick if I look up. I have just vomited all over my new red corduroy jumper.

I swallow hard and try to still my rumbling stomach. Not daring to look toward the overwhelming ceiling, I keep my eyes on the floor and murmur, "I can wait, you swim."

Not waiting to hear more, Penny dives into the water and begins vigorous breast strokes toward the opposite end of the pool. Back and forth, back and forth, she glides through the green water with astonishing speed. I watch drearily for a while, then bow my head and shut my eyes. I struggle not to be sick again and finally fall asleep.

I awake to hear Penny say, "Ruth, wake up! We have to hurry and get you in the tub before dinner. I have a tennis game at seven o'clock." To my surprise, Penny doesn't say a word during the trip back to Ivy Hall. The hot bathwater relaxes and soothes me. How good it is to be clean.

When I am out of the tub, Penny speaks. "Ruth, why don't you put your pajamas and robe on now? I'll bring your dinner back to you before my tennis game. It'll be so much easier for both of us."

A lump forms in my throat and tears find their way down my cheeks as I stammer, "B . . . b . . . but tonight is the welcoming dinner for freshmen. I want to go!"

"Ruth, you have to realize right now you can't attend every social function at college. In fact, with my five phys ed courses, swim meets, and tennis tournaments, you will be lucky if you attend eight o'clock classes once a week. Tonight I cannot take you to the dinner because I have a game." Then she adds, "I wonder why I took this job!"

That evening Penny brings me a tray with cold fried chicken, cold scalloped potatoes, and cold eggplant. This is not the only meal I eat in my room. During the first week, I eat only one of twenty-one meals in the dining room.

My dorm fast becomes a prison. I get out of it only when Penny takes me to class. Tension builds in me steadily, and my right ankle cramps and bends whenever I stand up. Penny is irritated when my foot takes ten to thirty seconds to relax before I can take a step.

As we enter our room on Wednesday evening after the sport orientation banquet, my ankle tenses and turns. I start to fall and almost pull Penny down with me. She catches herself, yanks me upright, and throws me on my bed two feet away. I begin to cry.

"Stop crying, you big baby! I haven't hurt you." Coming close to me, she wags a finger in my face. "I'm telling you this much, Ruth Webb, I'm not taking any more nonsense from you. Tomorrow morning I'm going to see the dean."

I don't sleep much that night. We rise at seven o'clock. Penny buttons my dress and ties my shoes without comment. She goes to the cafeteria for breakfast and, after twenty minutes, returns with orange juice, toast, and coffee.

Noisily plunking down the tray and shoving my chair so near the desk that I can hardly breathe, my roommate announces, "I'm off to see Dean Gillette. I'll let you know what we decide when I come back."

The door is halfway shut when she opens it again and says over her shoulder, "Don't worry, Ruth, I'll pack your things to go home." My throat suddenly is dry and I can hardly eat. My stomach cramps and refuses the food.

What is Penny telling the dean? I wonder fearfully. Minutes tick by . . . then an hour . . . an hour and a half. My cramps grow to crisis status. I have to go to the bathroom. Quick! I grab the crab, my trusty three-legged cane, which is fortunately standing beside the desk. I walk as fast as I can, and I get there just in time.

Then Penny bursts in, followed closely by a tall, slender, gray-haired woman. "Ruth," Penny says, "Dean Gillette is here to tell you her plans for you."

"Ruth," Dean Gillette smiles as she sits down, "Penny tells me that she can't take care of you. You require too much of her time. She has a heavy course load and a busy sports schedule."

I look at Dean Gillette and then at the red-faced Penny. I open my mouth to say, "She really doesn't spend much time at all with me," but the words won't come.

The dean continues, "I've called your parents and we have made an agreement allowing you to stay in college, at least for this year. You will have this room as your private domain."

"Who will help me?" I interrupt.

"Mrs. McGinty from the kitchen has consented to come in every morning and evening to help you bathe and dress. She will bring your meals in to you."

"How do I get to classes?" I ask.

"I'm asking freshmen to escort you to and from your classes and to the library. Now how about it, is it worth a trial?" the dean inquires gravely.

My need for a college degree to obtain a self-supporting job helping others flashes across my mind.

I swallow hard and say, "Yes, I'll try it. I want a college education."

The dean smiles. "Ruth, you've made a wise decision," she says. "And here comes Mrs. McGinty."

In walks a rather plump, middle-aged lady with sparse, carrot red hair and watery blue eyes. This good-natured soul is destined to be my faithful helper throughout the school year.

Mrs. McGinty not only takes care of me, cleans my room, and punctually brings me three meals a day but also she proceeds to fatten me up. Day after day, she brings me creamy soups, rich casseroles, ice cream, and pies. I obey her injunctions to "eat up" and soon weigh 105 pounds—more than I've ever weighed.

Above and beyond her loving concern for my health, Mrs. McGinty is the spirit guide who enables me to take the first year of my college education at Angel. She is one of many persons whom I later call spirit guides, people who continually come into my life at the right time and in the right way.

I settle into a rather humdrum existence at Angel College—sleeping, dressing, eating, classes, and homework for my courses—

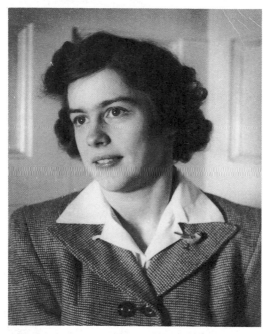

Ruth Cameron Webb, age twenty-one, a first-year student at Angel College

the English Bible, Freshman English, American History, Sociology, and Hygiene. I almost never see any of my classmates, only when they walk me to class. I rarely attend social events in the evening. The radio is my only source of entertainment and connection with the world outside my room.

On Sunday afternoons I listen to services from Philadelphia's inner-city churches. That day I listen to four hours of fundamentalist pleading, "Accept Jesus and be saved!" This experience clinches once and for all my rejection of the exclusive and simplistic doctrine of literalism. Dad's frequent visits and weekends at home provide sanity-preserving relief. In fact, my father plays a large part in helping me confront one aspect of my disability.

During Mother's visit to her sister, I write Dad and ask him to buy me a formal dress for the autumn dance. Dad answers with a very loving and tactful note. He writes, "Your handicap makes it 'socially impossible' for you to attend the dance. Your mother and I love you too much to allow you to enter such embarrassing situations. Don't worry, Pilikia, there will be other affairs at which you will shine."

At first, I am deeply hurt but the longer I think about Dad's letter, the more I agree that he is right. With my grimacing face and hard-to-understand speech, what business do I have attending a college dance? My parents' old question—"what will people think?"—pops up again. I spend many nights pondering this matter.

Two of my classmates offer to walk me on-and-offstage during the yearly song contest. I step up onstage without difficulty and stand between two classmates throughout our performance.

When we are finished, my friends include me in the exit march. They each grab an arm and hustle me down the two hundred feet of the auditorium. My whole body tenses and my right ankle turns so that my foot resembles a golf club. Every step brings shooting pains ascending from my bent ankle up the back of my leg to my hip. Sweat pours down my cheeks and I pant noisily. Dad later describes the spectacle by saying, "They sure gave you a bum's rush!"

In some eerie way, that traumatic event casts a piercing searchlight upon the part of myself which I try to ignore, my physical disability. Whenever I think of my march down that aisle, I am embarrassed and disgusted, and I yearn to be someone else.

Often I wonder why God allowed me to be injured at birth. Have I done anything to deserve cerebral palsy? Why can't I walk and talk like everybody else?

That stumble down the aisle undoubtedly shortens my career at Angel College. My grades are good—three A's and two B's. However, this doesn't forestall my dismissal. In a hastily arranged interview the next day, Dean Gillette icily informs my parents and me that she has decided I am too handicapped to stay at Angel for another year. She adds, "Your classmates have complained about the never-ceasing task of taking you to and from classes." She then shuts off the discussion by stating flatly, "Mrs. McGinty is retiring in June, and there will be no one available to help you next year."

"Well," mutters Dad, "we'll just have to find another college, won't we, Pilikia? It will take time but we'll find one—the right one this time." He pats my shoulder. I nod while tears run down my cheeks. Mother turns away but not before I see her eyes are overflowing.

So home I go for another dreary year, during which one long boring day stretches into the next. I sit in my upstairs room again and look down on the busy traffic below. I think wearily, I am nineteen years old. Every one but me has a place to go and something to do.

Dad sees that I get to the movies, to church, and on long car rides with him. On these rides, we sit side by side in the front seat, sometimes for hours without saying a word. Many thoughts pass between us. I feel his many frustrations with his career disappointments and his deep remorse that I, his only daughter, am crippled for life. At these times, he sighs. Then I smile, and we revel in each other's love. He reaches for my hand and grips it hard.

Dad is very clever with his hands. He is happiest when he is fixing a dripping faucet or repairing a light switch for Mother. Then his great need to be appreciated is satisfied.

One afternoon, Dad brings up my future by saying, "Pilikia, your mother and I have been thinking about your vocational plans. We want to find a college where you can earn your bachelor's degree. I want you to get a master's degree, perhaps a Ph.D. You'll never be satisfied unless you can support yourself, and judging from my experience, you won't be able to get and hold a job without a doctorate. Are you willing to try, Pilikia?"

As I slowly nod my head, Dad reaches over and squeezes my hand. "That's my girl," he murmurs proudly. "Remember your old motto: If at first you don't succeed, try, try again. Say, what have you decided to take as your college major?"

"I really don't know, Dad. I want to take something I can use to get a job." I sigh and add, "And I want to help people."

"Why don't you take modern languages to prepare to be a translator? You already read French well, and you can add Spanish and German to your repertoire. Your handicap won't hinder this vocational choice."

"That's an idea. I'll think about it," I say uncertainly.

The winter drags wearily on. The fresh bright colors of spring finally come. They comfort me, and at the same time, my chest throbs with pain. How can nature be so beautiful when I am so miserable? Will I ever get a college degree and be able to support myself?

One day in early May, Aunt Ethel comes in with practical surprises—an apron for Mother, a screwdriver for Dad, a new stamp issue for David, and a blue smock for me to wear when I eat.

She suddenly asks, "Ruth, have you found another college yet?"

"No," I answer sadly. "I don't think any school will take me."

"Have you thought of Drew University in Madison, New Jersey? It's where Uncle Harold's father, John Underwood Faulkner, the famous theologian, taught for many years."

"No," I murmur.

"Then why don't you write for their catalog and an application to the college?" queries my aunt, looking at Dad.

"We'll do that right now!" exclaims my Dad.

Friday brings an application and catalog from Drew. I see that the required courses are much like those of any other college. I sigh and think, What's the use of trying?

Dad makes me help him fill out the application. After answering two pages of questions, we come to the last question: "Do you have a physical handicap?"

Dad looks at me and says, "What shall we put down?"

"Cerebral palsy, I suppose. Oh Dad, they'll never take me!"

"You won't know that if you don't finish the application and mail it," asserts my father. "Here, sign on the bottom line." I oblige, and Dad puts it in Friday's mail.

The next Thursday I receive a letter from Dean Bradshaw of

Drew University inviting me to come for an interview the following Wednesday. Although I try hard not to expect Drew to accept me, I look forward to the visit with great eagerness.

So, on a sunny May day, Mother, Dad, and I drive the hundred miles to Madison, New Jersey, pass under a carved stone arch, and park at a long brick building with a tall white clock tower.

Inside we enter the dean's office and are greeted by a smiling secretary, who says, "You must be the Webbs Dean Bradshaw is expecting." She leads us into a large, comfortable room which looks out on a woods filled with giant oak trees.

"You are looking at Drew Forest." A smiling man rises and shakes hands with each of us. "I'm Dean Bradshaw."

When we are seated, he says, "Your application states you are related to our noted church historian, John Underwood Faulkner."

"Very distantly," says Dad. "He was my brother-in-law's father."

"Well," asserts the Dean. "He's well remembered at Drew. If Miss Webb comes to Drew, she'll probably live in Professor Faulkner's old residence."

Turning to me, he says, "Miss Webb, I see from your transcript that you have twenty-nine credits—and all A's and B's. We can accept all these credits. If you come to Drew, what will be your major?"

"Modern languages, Sir," I reply. "I hope to be a translator."

"Do you intend to work for the government?"

"I'll work wherever I can get a job," I murmur fervently.

"I like your spirit!" exclaims the Dean. "I think you'll be a good Drew student. But can you take care of yourself and care for your daily needs? How will you get from place to place around campus?"

Here Dad intervenes. "We are willing to pay a student to room with Ruth. Do you have a young woman who would be willing to help her in return for payment of her tuition?"

"Hmm . . ." The Dean thinks out loud. "Perhaps. We do have a young lady who may be interested. I'll see her tomorrow, and if she is willing to help you, I'll recommend that the Admissions Committee accept you as a freshman with advanced standing for the summer term. The committee meets this Friday morning. I will telephone you that afternoon and let you know their decision. By that time I should know if we can find a roommate for you."

Thursday takes a long time to pass, and Friday morning just inches by. After lunch I sit near the phone in anxious anticipation. What if the committee rejects me? What if no one wants to be my roommate?

Mother hurries by, a full dustpan in hand. "Don't give up the ship before you have even launched it, Ruthie," she remarks gently.

"Be patient a little while longer!" Just then the phone rings. A voice on the other end says, "This is Dean Bradshaw. Is Miss Ruth Webb there?"

"You are speaking with her," I breathe.

"Hello, Miss Webb. I have the honor to inform you that the Admissions Committee approved your application to enter Drew in July. Miss Bonnie Appleton, an exceptionally caring young lady, has agreed to be your assistant this summer in return for her $300-a-term tuition."

"We can manage that," Mother says, speaking on her bedroom extension.

Before Drew's summer term opens, my brother, David, graduates from high school with honors on D-Day, June 6, 1944, the beginning of the end of World War II in Europe. He then enrolls for his freshman year at Wesleyan University in New Haven, Connecticut.

On a hundred-degree Saturday in July, Dad drives me to Drew. We park in front of a whitewashed brick building and see a sign with big gold letters, FAULKNER HOUSE. The front door opens before Dad and I reach it, and a pretty young woman with short dark hair and smiling blue eyes greets us.

"You must be Ruth Webb and her dad. Come right in. I'm Marie Frataloni, head resident of Faulkner House. Your roommate, Bonnie Appleton, is unpacking. Come and meet her."

Bonnie opens the door and gives me a big hug as she says, "Ruth, you're here at last. We're going to have lots of fun living in Faulkner House this summer."

The first summer at Drew is indeed a wonderful time. I take three courses—History of Social Thought, Heredity, and General Psychology. The next term, when I continue French, I realize I cannot speak French but can only read it. I don't think I can be a translator without speaking the language. I will have to give up that ambition.

On the other hand, psychology professor James McClintock holds me spellbound. I soon decide that my major will be psychology instead of modern languages. I am very sure that my psychology major under Dr. McClintock will prepare me to help people.

I now turn to Dr. Mac for guidance and request that he accept me as a psychology major. I very much like the prospect of majoring in psychology, so I am overjoyed when Dr. Mac accepts me as an advisee. Throughout my years at Drew, he is my teacher, counselor, and friend.

It does not take Dr. Mac long to sense my frustration about my disability. He suggests that I meet with him to talk over some of my problems, and I begin my first psychotherapy sessions with him.

During the next two and a half years, my major professor and I explore many subjects revolving around my feelings of inferiority and unworthiness. He never belittles the inner and outer problems created by my cerebral palsy, but he challenges me to look beyond them and to design realistic life goals.

Chief among these problems are deep feelings of inferiority and anger about my cerebral palsy. Again and again these questions reverberate in my mind: Why am *I* handicapped? Why won't anyone give me a job? Am I good for nothing? Can I never help people and support myself? With Dr. Mac's aid, I begin to recognize and acknowledge these feelings.

My vocational future is a crucial issue. It seems a hopeless task to find a school or institution that will even think of "hiring the handicapped," to say nothing of a woman with cerebral palsy. My persevering professor writes letter after letter to government and private agencies seeking leads on job opportunities for me. He receives many polite answers, but not one offers me a job.

Dr. Mac is my lifelong spirit guide. During the three years he seeks a job for me, he never lets me give up thinking there is a job somewhere for me. This hope quiets my anxiety about the future and enables me to enjoy my Drew days to the nth degree.

Those Drew days pass quickly—attending classes, studying in the library, writing papers, and taking tests, as well as participating in unexpected and funny events.

One such event occurs on a cold January evening, when my roommate and I are the only ones ascending the thirty-five marble stairs leading to the second floor of the library. I am wearing my thick mouton fur coat (a present from Aunt Louise), which makes me feel like Winnie the Pooh caught in the honey jar.

As we near the top step, Bonnie loses her grip on my wrist for a second, and in trying to regain her grasp, she grabs my coat instead. Her hold does not prevent me from falling, and with my fur coat forming a protective skin from my neck to my knees, I roll over and over all the way down the stairs. I am not hurt and I begin to giggle. By the time I reach the bottom, I am laughing so hard, I can't answer Bonnie for several minutes. Forever after that evening, we refer to the library staircase as the Drew rolling coaster.

As a member of the Drew Fellowship, one day I am invited to write a presentation for one of the college chapel services. I choose Jesus's parable of the talents and emphasize our obligation to use our talents to help others. Afterward I doubt very much that my message is worth anything, but Dr. Mac's assurance that my words are an honest reflection of my wish to serve people makes me happy.

I begin to write feature articles for the *Drew Acorn*, the weekly campus newspaper. My subjects range from the noisy clatter of the metal trays in the dining room (inherited from the Navy V-12 program) to the debate about the Saturday night curfew for freshmen girls. My three years at Drew pass very quickly. Although most of the time is spent in classes, studying in the library, or typing papers in my room, fun times do occur. I see plays by Shakespeare, Eugene O'Neill, and Tennessee Williams.

At Faulkner House parties, I listen to chatter about what young man is asking what Faulknerite to the spring prom. I never dream of getting such an invitation. However, in my sophomore year at Drew, Charles Chrismeyer, a tall, blond preministerial student, not only goes through a very formal ceremony to ask me to the prom but also buys me my first corsage, an enormous lavender and yellow orchid. I am thrilled!

This time Mother is home, and in contrast to Dad's negative reaction to my attending a boy-girl affair at Angel College, she springs into action. She buys me a powder blue, silk evening dress with a wide collar and puffed sleeves. Almost as excited as I, she then drives the hundred miles to bring me the wonderful dress. I wear a blue velvet choker, black slippers, and Mother's pink-flowered Chinese shawl. Bonnie sets my hair and helps me dress. "You're a real Cinderella! You'll wow Charles!" she declares.

Charles and I have a lovely time. We sit on the east side of the gym and chat. He tells funny stories and feeds me sandwiches and innumerable chocolate cupcakes. I am on top of the world. This night is never-to-be-forgotten.

As Bonnie graduates two years before I do, I have to find another roommate. Davis Conrad, a psychology junior, agrees to help me. A "women's libber" far in advance of the sixties, Davis moves into my room and my life with an armful of books, proclaiming, "Ruth, if we're going to be roommates, you must know I sleep nude."

Davis is quite unlike any one I have ever met. Her parents have taught her not to be afraid of being unconventional. As a result, Davis takes pleasure in being avant-garde. She likes to try new things—new hairdos, new low-neck dresses, new ways of playing bridge. She even raises snails in a tin cracker box on the bay windowsill.

One Saturday after lunch, Davis says to me, "Ruth, how come you fall a lot and don't get hurt?"

I laugh. "Oh, they made me fall on a mattress before they taught me to walk."

"Can you teach me to fall?" Davis asks.

"Sure, let me show you," I respond, as I move to the center of our wide room.

I intend to demonstrate to my roommate how to relax before falling, but Davis decides to fall at the same time I do. My head hits her cheekbone just below her left eye. For two weeks thereafter, Davis sports an enormous black eye. When asked if she has been hit with a knee or fist, she replies with alacrity, "Head!"

Next year, in the spring of 1947, the black civil rights movement is just coming to life. On the evening of the Faulkner House spring party, Davis meets Rob Dunlap, a soft-spoken and deeply intelligent man whose skin is a beautiful chocolate brown. From then until June commencement, when the three of us graduate, Davis and Rob are inseparable. Their occasional strolls in the little town of Madison bring call after call to the dean from enraged townsfolk.

Davis and Rob ignore the storm around them. Their future is securely planned. They marry soon after commencement, and after earning Ph.D.'s, they settle in Hawaii. Rob teaches at the University of Hawaii and becomes well known for his research in learning processes. Davis is a successful psychotherapist and mother of four. Whenever I think of them, this dauntless pair gives me courage to persist on my own journey.

Senior comprehensive exams are given two weeks before June commencement. The nearer the time comes, the more panicky I become. If I don't pass, I won't graduate. If I don't get a B on the comps, I won't graduate *cum laude*. This goal now seems to be of earth-shaking importance. It will help me prove to unbelievers that I can compete.

The afternoon before the exams, I get nervous and begin to cry. Davis tries to comfort me by saying, "Don't cry, Ruth. I know so much depends on how well we do tomorrow, but we have been over the review material a hundred times. It's time for a break. I'll call Rob and suggest we all go downtown to the diner. Are you up to being gawked at?"

I reply, "I've been gawked at by experts!"

Rob agrees without hesitation. Pretty soon he and Davis are walking arm in arm while they both push my wheelchair. I feel the focus of hostile eyes as we enter the diner and sit at a table. This unfriendly surveillance continues as we order and consume cheeseburgers and coffee. Rob and Davis appear not to notice their audience as they discuss plans for the summer.

When we are outside again, I look back at Rob and Davis and say, "Do people always stare at you like that?"

Davis smiles. "Yep," she says. "Somehow we never lack an audience."

Then I'm not the only side show, I think.

After breakfast the next morning, Davis runs over to the dean's office to see if the comps results are posted. Five minutes later she bursts into our room crying, "Ruth, we all passed! You and I got B's and Rob got an A."

I send a thank-you heavenward. Now I will get my degree *cum laude* in June of 1948. Joyful exultation fills me: Let people gawk— I'll be an A.B. *cum laude*!

The week after comps, Dr. Mac arranges a job interview for me with Dr. Richard Odorf of the U.S. Office of Vocational Rehabilitation in Washington, D.C. My former roommate, Bonnie, agrees to take a day off from her hospital job and accompany me on the train.

At the Vocational Rehabilitation office, we are ushered into a small booth.

"Hello, Miss Webb. I'm Rich Odorf, rehabilitation counselor. I understand you're from Drew University and looking for a job with the government. What is your training? What kind of job are you seeking?" His questions come with machine-gun rapidity.

"I'll take any job where I can use my psych background," I say. Dr. Odorf looks at my papers. "You have excellent grades, but since you have just an A.B. degree, I can offer you only an entry-level job as a counselor intern in Social Security. There you would be registering pension applicants. Does this position interest you?"

"What would be Ruth's top position and salary?" Bonnie queries.

"Well, after five years, she might possibly become a district supervisor with a salary of $20,000 to $30,000," Dr. Odorf declares. Turning to me, he asks, "Miss Webb, are you interested?"

"Y . . . y . . . yes," I say hesitantly. "But I am hoping for more of a counseling job."

"My dear young lady!" exclaims Dr. Odorf. "Be realistic! You have such severe speech and ambulation problems that few employers will hire you. Take what I offer you while it is available. It may not be here tomorrow."

"May I let you know? I'd like to think about it. Thank-you very much for your offer."

Dr. Odorf rises from his desk and shakes hands with first me and then Bonnie. As he walks out the door, he mutters loudly, "A sad case. Too much education for such a physical handicap."

Bonnie and I look at each other. Then she says softly, "Ruth, you know you're always going to meet people who can't picture you as a helping professional. They believe you should always be on the receiving end of any aid."

I muse on her words as I sit in my heavy, iron wheelchair, waiting for the six-o'clock train to arrive. Gradually my spirits rise as I think about all the exams I have passed and papers I have written the past three years. And now I'm about to graduate *cum laude*. Surely I will get a job with this record.

These rosy thoughts are interrupted by a little girl, perhaps ten years old, who holds out her hand and shyly drops a quarter in my lap. My pink daydream suddenly turns black, and anger reddens my face.

I think, Who does she think I am? Can't she see I'm a big college senior, ready to graduate next week? Why is she treating me like a beggar?

Indignation runs hot throughout my body as I grab the quarter with Lefty and hurl it about ten feet from me. Surprise and fear register on the child's face, and she quickly disappears.

I later learn that I have been caught in an "overlapping situation," an uncomfortable experience that occurs when any person, with or without a disability, is treated in a manner inferior to his or her accustomed role.

Throughout the year, Dr. Mac has been urging me to consider earning a master's degree. "There are not many jobs for even non-handicapped persons with just A.B. degrees," he often warns.

So I apply to three big-name graduate schools—New York Teachers College, New York University, and the University of Iowa. I have the distinction of being turned down by all three.

The week before commencement, Dean Bradshaw calls me in to his office. "Ruth," he begins, "Professor McClintock tells me you are having trouble getting into graduate school. I have taken the liberty of telling the chancellor of Syracuse University about you. He is a former dean of Drew. He has asked Dr. Crusen, chairman of the Special Education Department, to take you as an advisee."

The dean hesitates, then proceeds. "Dr. Crusen has agreed to accept you on condition that he not be responsible for helping you get a job. He doesn't think that people with cerebral palsy should—"

"Work with other people," I supply. "I've heard that opinion before!"

"Dr. McClintock and I are counting on you to change that view. The important thing for you now is to get the training you need to enter a helping profession. Will you accept Dr. Crusen's offer?" the dean queries earnestly.

I think a minute. I may never have another chance to go to grad school.

To Dean Bradshaw I murmur, "Yes, I accept."

"Fine!" exclaims the dean. "I'll call him right away."

The week rapidly passes, and commencement day looms dark and showery. I hope against hope the sun will shine by 2:00 P.M. Alas, it rains at 1:30. Dean Bradshaw regretfully orders that the ceremony be held in the refectory chapel. This is my first disappointment which the long-anticipated day brings.

That morning Dr. Mac gently but firmly tells me that to avoid any embarrassment (caused by my awkwardness in climbing up and down the stage steps), a classmate will bring my degree to me.

I am so upset over this second disappointment that I begin to cry when the university president starts to confer our degrees. I have waited so long to accept my degree and shake the president's hand. Now that moment will never come.

The small chapel overflows with seniors, faculty, and parents. It is hot and humid. I am sweating, and my black gown clings to my back. Someone hands me a wet paper towel to wipe my face and whispers, "Don't cry, Ruth! It will soon be over."

Soon over. Yes, all the happy days, busy with meaning are gone. I think, Now stretching endlessly before me are days and days at home or the Antlers, filled with boredom. No friends, no studies, no job.

Commencement is indeed soon over, leaving few memory traces except my diploma, engraved on a real sheepskin. Mother, Dad, Dave, and Aunt Louise gather around to congratulate me.

"Pilikia, you did it! You showed the unbelievers!" shouts Dad as he hugs me.

Mother bends low and kisses me. "You've made it, Sweetie!" she says.

Dave just grins.

Aunt Louise, who never finished college, kisses me and whispers, "Ruth, now that you have one degree, I hope you're satisfied. Getting another degree is a foolish idea. You'd never use it."

I start to defend my education and career hopes but smile when I remember Dr. Mac's farewell words: "Ruth, we got you into graduate school. Now it's up to you to become a real pro."

My usually matter-of-fact professor had softly added, "Anyone as determined as you are to help others will eventually create her own role to serve humanity."

I look at my dear ones around me, and then I spy Dr. Mac a little way down the refectory stairs.

I wonder, Who is right in predicting my future? Aunt Louise or Dr. Mac? Can it be that I'm the one to answer that question?

With a flash of momentary reverence for these self-sufficient college days, I add, With God's help!

5

Graduate School and the Journey Beyond

It is September 15, 1948, and Dad and I are standing before a long registration table in the noisy Syracuse University gym.

"So you are Miss Webb! I've heard a lot about you." A tall slender man with piercing black eyes greets me. "I am Dr. Crusen, your advisor and chairman of the Special Education Department. Have you spoken to the dean of women about your room assignment?"

"Yes," I answer. "She has given me a big, sunny suite of rooms with two roommates to help me."

My new advisor continues, "I understand you are seeking a master's degree in clinical psychology. Would you consider a double major and add special education to clinical psychology? This will give you courses in clinical psych and still permit me to be your advisor."

I look at Dad, standing beside me. He nods and then I agree. Special ed isn't what I want, but it will aid me to help people.

The professor continues, "Your courses in special ed will cover aphasia, audiology, and orthopedic handicaps. Clinical psych will acquaint you with mental disorders and counseling theories. You are also required to take three education courses. I presume you will take comprehensive examinations rather than write a master's thesis."

"Yes, Sir," I reply.

Then Dr. Crusen looks at me quizzically and says, "Miss Webb, I trust you know I'm accepting you as my advisee under protest. The chancellor of the university has ordered me to do so. I will make no effort to place you in a job. I don't think your handicap will allow you to join the educational or psychological professions."

This time I do not answer but think, Sir, I'm going to prove you wrong.

Throughout my time at SU, Dr. Crusen keeps this promise. Although he is always polite and helpful in arranging my class schedules and extremely fair in grading my work, job placement is a taboo subject. When a fellow student suggests that I get some practical experience by helping in Dr. Crusen's c.p. clinic, my unyielding professor indignantly rejects her idea.

Dr. Crusen advocates the theory that brain-injured persons are distracted by individual details in their environment. They see, hear, and feel objects and people around them as many separate stimuli, rather than integrating them into "related wholes."

At the time I don't realize how much I threaten Dr. Crusen. My presence in his classes so unnerves Dr. Crusen that many years later he cites me in a book as an example of a brain-injured person who is "overeducated."

(There comes a time, years later, when I disprove his theory. While working in Wisconsin, I attend one of Dr. Crusen's lectures and introduce myself as a rehabilitation counselor. His amazed face gives me immense satisfaction.)

Dr. Hann, who teaches both phenomenology and nondirective

counseling, is a great contrast to Dr. Crusen. Soft-spoken and gentle, he practices the theory he teaches. He asserts that the way one thinks and feels about oneself at a given moment determines one's behavior at that moment.

To get acquainted with his students and to help them explore their self-attitudes, Dr. Hann requires each class member to write a one-page "reaction report" every week. In this way we learn about ourselves and Dr. Hann comes to know us very well.

The first day of class, Dr. Hann announces that he will not grade our work; each of us can best evaluate what he or she has learned. He will meet with each student to discuss whether he or she has earned an A or B.

One morning, as I wait for Maria, my roommate, to help me to the next class, Dr. Hann comes and sits beside me. "Miss Webb," he says, "what do you think your grade should be, A or B?"

I hesitate and have a sudden insight. Until now I really haven't understood that Dr. Hann is not only teaching us that perception determines behavior. He is also showing us that each student is the one who best knows what he or she has learned from the course. I look at my prof and say, "Dr. Hann, it took all semester for me to understand that you really trust us to rely on our own perceptions. I'm a slow learner, but I won't forget this lesson. I think I deserve a B."

Dr. Hann smiles. "Well, so be it. You have your B."

In counseling class, Dr. Hann adheres strictly to the principles of nondirective psychotherapy, as espoused by his famous teacher, Carl Rogers. Time and again he exhorts his counselors-to-be, "Listen to your clients with your whole being. Reflect their feelings. Clarify their words. But don't interpret. Don't verbalize your judgments. There's always a possibility your understanding of the problem is not correct and that your too-directive interpretations can stir up serious, perhaps catastrophic, problems."

Dr. Hann makes a lasting impression on me. He teaches me not only to trust my own feelings and thoughts and to act upon them but also to heed the feelings and thoughts of those around me. By the time the course ends, I feel so well versed in nondirective psychotherapy that I request and receive an A.

That summer I take a workshop on cerebral palsy, little dreaming of its traumatic climax. The class includes thirty-nine professionals, all trainers of c.p. children.

One morning Miss O'Neil, the nurse instructor suddenly asks me, "Ruth, will you demonstrate to the class how you move your wheelchair at our final meeting this afternoon? Dr. Phelps, the famous cerebral palsy specialist from Baltimore, will be here to lecture. I want you to show the class what an adult c.p. can do after early training."

I hesitate and think. I hate to display my awkward movements before a crowd. I get so tense. But then, perhaps my demonstration will help people understand cerebral palsy better.

"All right," I say. "Dr. Phelps is an old friend. I'll do it for him."

It is a most eventful afternoon. Dr. Phelps stands on a wide stage about two feet high and gives a short lecture on the three most common types of cerebral palsy. He then demonstrates the pathological muscle patterns exhibited by each type on three youngsters.

When Dr. Phelps's demonstrations are over, our instructor introduces me with these words: "Your classmate, Ruth Webb, has had many years of training with Dr. Phelps and has achieved much independence in daily living skills. She will show us how she uses her feet and her good left arm to move her wheelchair."

Miss O'Neil takes me up the short ramp on the left side of the stage and whispers, "Go to it, Ruth! Show them what you can do."

As I look at my fellow students, their faces blur and I begin to sweat. Lefty grabs the wheel handle and moves it ahead. My chair turns toward the right, toward the edge of the stage. I quickly put my left foot forward, and the chair again faces the right curtain. I repeat these movements again and again. It seems an eternity before I reach the end of the gauntlet of staring faces. Panting and sweating, I finally near the far side of the stage.

Miss O'Neil puts her arm around my shoulders and says, "Thank-you, Ruth, for showing us your courageous persistence. It's a lesson we shall all remember."

My grades for the summer term include an A for my performance at the cerebral palsy workshop. I chuckle as I exclaim, "Four A credits. I sure earned them!"

The cerebral palsy workshop ends my studies at SU. I do not attend the fall graduation. I receive my master's degree by mail at the Antlers in early September 1949, before the family returns to Swarthmore. Now the burning question of my future can no longer be ignored. What will I do now? Will I ever have a chance to support myself?

One morning late in October, Mother hears about a wonderful speech correction center on the Dorothy Kilgallen radio show. Located in Prairie Village, Kansas, in the center of the United States, the Institute for Better Speech is designed to "study and correct speech defects."

Mother and Dad are quite excited about the possibility that my speech can be improved. Within a week, Mother, Dad, and I drive to White Plains, New York, for an entrance interview.

A man with broad shoulders attached to a rugged frame, a friendly smile, and the largest hands I've ever seen greets us. "Hello, Mr. and Mrs. Webb and Ruth. I'm Dr. Martin Bush from the Institute for Better Speech. Let's see what your speech problems are and what we can do to help you communicate better."

He begins to test my articulation of first the vowels and then the consonants and their combinations. He notes that I do not raise my tongue tip to produce the sound l and I have difficulty with the soft th and str combinations. Dr. Bush remarks that my poor breath control forces me to take in air after every three or four words and contributes to the uneven pitch of my voice. "I think we can improve your breathing patterns and articulation as well as your voice quality," he declares. "How about coming to us after Christmas? In our new apartments, you can either live independently with two other young women or you can enter our housemother program."

Dad inquires with concern, "How much will all this cost?"

"Speech therapy three times a week costs $150 a month. Living independently costs $140, or $150 with a housemother. This makes the total cost around $550 a month."

Dad and Mother look at each other. She clears her throat and says, "We can manage it. I still am selling *My Bookhouse for Children*. I'll do anything I can to improve Ruth's speech."

When Dr. Bush suggests that I fly to Prairie Town on February first, Dad is startled. "Fly? Ruth can't fly unattended, can she?"

Dr. Bush smiles. "Our trainees come alone by plane from all over the world," he declares. "Don't be afraid to let Ruth travel alone. The airlines will take good care of her."

Mother turns to me excitedly. "Don't you have a friend from Angel College who lives in Wichita? I bet she would meet you."

I think a minute. "Yes, Mother, it is Darlene O'Conner. I knew her as a classmate in hygiene class." I exclaim, "I'm sure she will meet me. Her phone number is in my address book." My call that evening assures me that my friend will be waiting for my arrival in Wichita.

Mother and Dad are very quiet as we drive to the Philadelphia airport on January 5, 1950. Dad parks the car and gets out my wheelchair. We walk slowly to the gate. It is an act of courage for my dear parents to entrust me to the boarding agent. Both hate to see their "little girl" (though she is 27 years old) leave on a plane for the faraway Midwest.

When I get off the plane in Wichita six hours later, my "Drew carriage" has already arrived and is waiting for me at the gate. Standing beside it is my smiling friend, Darlene. As soon as I am seated in my chair, her arms enfold me in a quick bear hug. "Ruth," she cries, "I'm so glad you're here. You're going to have a great time at the institute."

When we are in the car, Darlene says, "On our way to Prairie

Village, I will tell you my news. Last January I married the neatest guy, Sam, a news photographer for our daily newspaper, the *Wichita Eagle*." Here Darlene hesitates. "We have a three-month-old baby named Sally Ann, who has Down's syndrome. We have enrolled her for physical therapy and prespeech training at the Institute. They are teaching Sally Ann to suck, chew, and swallow. After following this home program for only six weeks, she is sucking and swallowing a four-ounce bottle of formula at every feeding."

I look at my twenty-five-year-old friend. Tears stream from her gentle brown eyes.

"Oh Ruth," she whispers, "I am determined to do everything possible to give my baby the same chance in life as any other child."

I whisper back, "In my experience, determined parents ultimately win."

We turn down a broad four-lane boulevard which leads to a long rectangular brick building. "This is our world-famous Institute for Better Speech," Darlene proclaims. "There is the clinic building."

We have barely parked the car before a sweet-faced lady with silvery hair greets us. "Hello, Darlene." Looking at me, she asks, "Are you Ruth Webb? Welcome to the institute! I am Mrs. Harriman, your speech teacher. I will ride with you to your apartment and introduce you to Joanna Filer and Kitty Zerben, who will live with you."

In response to Mrs. Harriman's soft knock, the door is opened by a girl with a longish face and thin body. A plump girl with dark hair stands behind the first one.

"Hello, Joanna and Kitty," greets Mrs. Harriman. "Here is your new apartment mate, Ruth Webb."

I live with Joanna and Kitty for eight months. Kitty is aphasic and is often at a loss for words. She is Joanna's assistant around the house and is quite helpful in setting the table and washing dishes. Joanna is our housekeeper and cook. Although her religion forbids her to eat meat, she obligingly prepares it for Kitty and me. She is a cheerful person, and we share many interests. Jo is always there when I need her, to help me out of the bathtub, to button a small button, or just to share my daily triumphs and frustrations. She is a real friend.

My thrice-weekly speech lessons commence the day after my arrival. A young male escort wheels me over to Mrs. Harriman's office in the clinic building. "Hello, Ruth. I've been waiting for you," says Mrs. Harriman. "Today we will review what sounds you mispronounce or are difficult for you to say. Then we will evaluate your breathing patterns and your voice quality. We will also record your speech today and every three months to give us an objective measure of your progress."

Before I leave, Mrs. Harriman says, "Your speech training program at the institute will be intensive and will require much time and effort on your part. I will give you homework to practice for one hour every day. Your progress will depend on how much you practice. You may come over here and listen to your speech on the mirrorphone. [This machine is a precursor to the modern tape recorder.] We also have a spirometer on which you can practice lengthening your breath by blowing a tiny ball up a calibrated glass tube."

Mrs. Harriman is interested not only in my speech but also in my development as a person. She spends much time conducting "personality training," in which she tries to smooth out my rough spots. Sometimes the rough spots are great surprises to me. One day she accuses me of being arrogant to the escorts. I think I have been very polite to them, and I indignantly deny the accusation. I know that Mrs. Harriman is trying to help me, but sometimes her personality training hits a little too near home.

Most of the time, Mrs. Harriman is very understanding and helpful. It is she who suggests that I help in the academic classroom. On my first day in the classroom, the teacher, Mrs. Brown, asks me to help fifteen-year-old Beth read from a first-grade primer. I try to have the girl sound out the words, but somehow letters and their sounds mean nothing to her.

Mrs. Brown then explains to me that Beth has aphasia, a learning disorder resulting from injury to the brain. Dr. Bush compares the condition to a battery whose incoming and outgoing messages are scrambled and advocates that aphasic children be taught to read by associating letter shapes with familiar objects, e.g., the letter *h* can be printed to resemble a straight-backed chair. I slowly learn how to teach aphasic children by illustrating the learning material with familiar objects.

In regard to new friends, I become quite attached to Hector, who refuses to tell me her real Hungarian name. She runs a beauty shop on the northern edge of the institute grounds. She adopts me as her Godchild and takes me shopping and to the doctor. She is always bringing me cakes, cookies, and candy, which she makes from recipes brought from Hungary. She certainly is one of my spirit guides. One day Hector brings me a six-month-old female puppy. She is a tan fox terrier with a white nose, chest, and paws. I call her Ginger, and we become very attached to each other. She is soon housebroken and quickly learns her name as well as the meaning of "no." The little dog becomes my constant companion.

My thoughtful dad has just sent me a three-wheeled twenty-inch tricycle. Knowing the trike can bring me new freedoms, I exert much effort to master my new riding machine. The back axle isn't wide enough to prevent the trike from tipping over when the front wheel is at right angles to the frame. The inevitable happens. One morning, when I try to turn around, I cut the front wheel too sharply and the trike falls with me still on the saddle. I incur a long bloody gash on the back of my head.

Mrs. Harriman happens to be at the door of the clinic building and sees me fall. She rushes out, picks me up, and takes me inside, where she washes and bandages my wound. Then she accompanies me on the ambulance trip to the hospital emergency room.

On the way home, she shakes her finger at me and delivers a lecture. "Ruth, if you would wear a helmet, you would not cut your head. Someday you will injure yourself very badly because of your foolish pride."

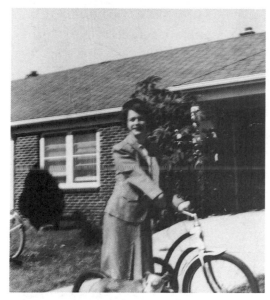

Ruth Cameron Webb, age twenty-six, with trike and dog Ginger in front of Ruth's apartment at the Institute for Better Speech, Prairie Village, Kansas

I look at Mrs. Harriman for a long time, and then I answer. "Mrs. Harriman, I would rather be injured physically than look more handicapped than I do. I want to be recognized as a person and not a spastic gimp!"

"But you are recognized as a person! Everyone here treats you as one, don't they?"

"You try living for one day as a c.p. and you'll see what I mean!" I retort.

Mrs. Harriman looks at me for a moment. Then she says quietly, "I know you have a hard role to play. You show us how to live with a handicap every day. If at times we seem to be rough on you, it's because we are trying to teach you to solve some of the personal and interpersonal problems your handicap creates." She takes my hand and says, "Don't be discouraged, and never, never give up—for your sake and for those who know and love you."

After my rear axle is broadened to thirty-two inches, I include

Ginger on my evening trike rides. Tied to the trike, she accompanies me around the four-block perimeter of the institute campus.

When my apartment mate, Joanna, finishes her training at the institute, Mrs. Harriman suggests that I go into the housemother program. To forestall this happening, I seek to try living alone in my apartment. The only help I request is to have lunch and dinner with Mrs. Malm, the housemother next door. Mrs. Harriman agrees, providing my parents consent. Mother and Dad readily give permission, and I start my two-week venture.

Meanwhile, Miss Aker, chief occupational therapist, teaches me ways to improve my dressing skills. I make a list of hurdles I must overcome if I'm to be entirely self-sufficient: fastening collar and cuff buttons as well as skirts, tying shoes, and applying lipstick.

In order to solve these problems, Miss Aker sews Velcro on the collars of my blouses as well as elastic on my cuffs. A loop of white tape under the waistband of my skirts permits Righty's forefinger to hold the button steady while Lefty maneuvers the hole around the button. I begin to use the one-bow knot that I learned at CRI again. Last but not least, Miss Aker makes a wooden holder for my lipstick and paints it red.

At the start of my two weeks alone, I rise at six o'clock to bathe, dress, get breakfast, and feed Ginger before leaving for the classroom at 8:45. During my time of independence, I reduce these three hours of preparation to one hour and fifteen minutes. I am thrilled!

My exaltation does not last long, for I soon learn how malicious gossip can destroy my self-confidence and that even my friends don't always believe that I am without blame.

Suddenly the air is filled with perplexing accusations. Mrs. Harriman, my revered teacher, tells me that she hears I am too self-centered and insist on my own way all the time. She hears that I routinely ask Joanna to tie my apron behind my back. She considers this to be a terrible fault!

When I vehemently deny these accusations, Mrs. Harriman does not believe me. I feel betrayed, and hot waves of shame and anger flood over me. Someone is lying about me. My integrity as a person is threatened.

Several days after this conversation, I look out the kitchen window and see Mrs. Malm seize Jerry, a deaf boy, by the shoulders and bang his head on the iron parallel bars again and again. I cannot believe my eyes.

I go to the phone, and after several misdialings by my tense fingers, I manage to get through to Mrs. Harriman. She can hardly believe my story but assures me that she will investigate it right away.

The inquiry does not take long. Mrs. Malm is fired and on her way home in two hours. Later, Mrs. Harriman comes to the apartment and thanks me profusely for reporting the incident. Offhandedly, she admits that Mrs. Malm is the source of the accusations against me.

Although I pass my two weeks of independent living with flying colors and even take care of my beloved dog, Mrs. Harriman convinces me that I will have more time and energy for speech training if I have a housemother. So, with a sigh I give up my new-found independence until another day. But now I know I can live alone.

My new housemother, Mrs. Bright, is a small lady who is a gentle soul, a widow of thirty years. Beneath her great timidity lies a tremendous eagerness to please. She seems very happy to cook and clean for me and Pam, my roommate from CRI days, who now shares my apartment. During the year and a half I live with Mrs. Bright, I grow to love her.

Whenever I think of Mrs. Bright, I see this picture. One night she wakes me up with a finger dripping blood on me and she whispers in a doleful voice, "Ruth, I broke the fan!" The fact that her finger is nearly severed is not important to Mrs. Bright. She is only concerned that I may be upset about the broken fan.

After visiting several churches, I join a friendly Congregational Church. Its members take turns driving me to services. George List,

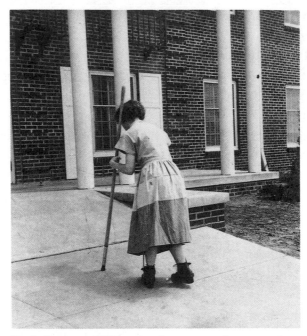

*Ruth Cameron Webb using four-pronged cane at the
Institute for Better Speech, c. 1950*

the minister, often visits me, and we have long talks about Jesus
and the church.

All this time I am walking back and forth the two hundred feet
from the apartment to the clinic building with the four-footed cane
which the institute carpenter made for me. This cane enables me
to walk to many places and enables me to get up from the floor. I
have more independence, but my walking is always slow and I fall
often.

When my falls become frequent and my head bears many scars
from half a dozen bloody wounds, April Bates, the physical therapist, decrees that I must wear a helmet. I become very adamant
that I will *not* wear the ugly thing because it will stigmatize me. I
refuse to discuss the matter with anyone. The more my friends urge
me to wear it, the more I insist that I will *not* wear a helmet.

Finally Dr. Perry, the institute physician, suggests I wear a little hat padded with cotton on the inside. I reluctantly agree, and Mrs. Bright buys a little red hat for me and lines it with heavy cotton. She pins it on my head with bobby pins. It does not prevent my head from being bumped, but it certainly saves me from almost daily lectures from my friends.

Meanwhile, I am having trouble teaching in the aphasic students' classroom. I just don't seem to be able to get through to my students. My self-confidence is so shattered by Mrs. Harriman's personality counseling that I cannot teach.

One day Mrs. Brown asks me if I would like to try teaching two students in a small room. I agree to try, and so wheelchair-bound Betty and tantrum- and seizure-wracked Trudy, both brain-injured and nonspeakers, become my special students.

As a motivational tool, I bring in a Sears catalog and large pieces of cardboard. I then group pictures of furniture according to rooms in a home. My students participate by pointing to the pictures and placing them in appropriate rooms.

Betty and Trudy very much enjoy this activity and are busy working every time Mrs. Brown looks in the door window. She commends me highly, and Mrs. Harriman also compliments me for a job well done. My greatest thrill comes when Betty's mother thanks me for giving her twenty-five-year-old daughter a reason to get up in the morning.

In conjunction with working with the two aphasic students, I begin taking courses in education and speech correction at the University of Wichita. My practice teaching is done in the aphasic students' classroom with Mrs. Brown acting as my supervising teacher.

In this way I gain the background for a teacher's certificate in the state of Kansas. But when I am ready to apply for one, Mrs. Harriman discourages me. "Your handicap is too great," she says.

As time goes on, I am given other responsibilities—cataloguing the books in the small, children's library, editing the weekly house paper, and tutoring a nineteen-year-old boy in fourth-grade reading and math. The tutoring job is the most fun, and I get paid fifty cents an hour. Eddie gains a whole grade in reading and half a grade in math in six months.

Pleasing Mrs. Harriman becomes more difficult as my training lengthens into three years. She spends more and more time on my personality adjustment. Her usual approach is to confront me suddenly with some faux pas—a thoughtless word, a forgotten thank-you, a remark that sounded arrogant. All these grave errors have been reported to her by other staff members.

One day after such a lecture, I become very upset and slide into an impenetrable fog of anger. This has become a frequent occurrence as Mrs. Harriman presses my personality training. Again and again I reproach myself in a never-ending cycle of accusations and self-justifications: If only I hadn't made that remark! I was trying to thank him; Why should anyone care whether or not I attend the adult group meetings? I am *not* going to be tattled on by peers; Mrs. Harriman scolds me enough. Angry tears gush from me the way hot lava spurts from a volcano.

It is four days before I come out of the present fog, and then I am very depressed. My friend, Hector, tries to help me out of this un-reality. She takes me to her home and listens to my troubles. I am angry with Mrs. Harriman, with my unknown accusers, and most of all, with myself. This depressed state does not improve when Mrs. Harriman announces that the institute plans to send me home in September. My training period is up. The institute has given me all the help it can. It is time to make room for someone else who is in need of speech training.

I am desperate. I do not want to go home to sit and do nothing. I have gained so much independence at the institute, and I don't want to lose it. I frantically search for a way to stay at the institute.

It is at this low point that a previously unknown spirit guide visits me. One Sunday afternoon there is a knock at the door. I open it to see a smiling middle-aged lady, who says, "Would you like to go for a ride with me? A friend of mine tells me that you need to get out for a bit." I readily accept her offer, and she takes me out into the country for a two-hour ride. We begin to tell each other about ourselves.

She starts, "My name is Ann Whitfield. Today I just wanted to get out into green cornfields and breathe the fresh air and to meet someone new. I sense you are having a hard time right now. Do you want to talk about it?" She stops the car on a grassy knoll, and I tell her my woes.

After half an hour or so, she says, "Ruth, why don't you take the initiative and get a job on your own to show the institute that you really are independent? I think if you do that, Dr. Bush will give you some more training at the institute." I never see Ann again, and I wonder if my friend Darlene sent her. Anyway, I always think of her as my spirit guide for that afternoon.

When I get home, I act on her suggestion and call five print shops and ask if they need a proofreader. The fifth man agrees to hire me and to pay me twenty-five cents a page. I will earn $5 for every twenty pages I correct. Maybe I can earn $20 a week if I work fast enough. Mr. Powers sends me a short glossary of proofreading symbols, and I learn them without difficulty. Mr. Powers is satisfied with the first proofs I finish, and I am assured of my first job.

Mrs. Harriman looks at me quizzically when I tell her.

"Now may I stay longer at the institute?" I inquire with bated breath.

Mrs. Harriman answers gravely. "I will have to talk to Dr. Bush about this. You sure want to stay here!"

"Oh, yes!" I answer earnestly. "I want to continue to teach, to edit the 'Weekly Log,' to take more speech training, and most of all, to be independent."

When Dr. Bush hears that I have found a job, he grants me three more months at the institute. I get the impression that Dr. Bush and Mrs. Harriman are surprised and pleased that I got the job on my own initiative.

I work hard during those three months, with the added task of proofreading four legal-sized pages of newsprint every night—and I do earn $20 a week. This is a real triumph, and I know I am surely on the road to independence.

Then Mrs. Harriman gives me another blow. One day she tells me that the neighbors have been complaining about Ginger barking at night and that I will have to get rid of her. I am heartbroken, for I love that little spirit.

When he hears about this, Dad writes that he wants me to bring the dog home. He suggests that I find someone to keep Ginger until I go home. Once more Hector comes to my rescue and offers to keep my dog. I am sad to part with Ginger, even temporarily, but I am relieved that I can take her home.

The dreaded day for me to depart from the institute inevitably approaches. Mother comes out and spends three days talking with my instructors and watching me work in the classroom and in speech classes. In my last speech session, Mrs. Harriman urges me to practice my speech every day. She also recommends that I limit my slow walking to the house.

Taking a sleeping compartment for herself and putting Ginger in a kennel in the baggage car, Mother takes the train the day before I leave. That evening I attend a farewell party given by the c.p. social group. The next morning I catch the TWA plane to Chicago, then to Philadelphia, and home to Swarthmore. It is just before Christmas 1953, and I am now thirty years old.

It is good to be with Mother and Dad again, but it is Ginger who completes my homecoming. She has only been in our home for a day and a half, yet she seems to know who is boss in our house. My mother has already gotten through to the dog that she is to stay in the kitchen.

When I sit down on the living room sofa, Ginger runs from the kitchen, leaps on the couch, and runs not to me but to my mother. It is as if she is seeking permission from Mother to come to me on the couch. Mother grants her permission with a laugh, and Ginger runs over to me on the other end of the sofa and plops herself down on my lap. In this way, Ginger makes me feel that coming home is not the end of the world.

Later that night, I think hopefully about my future. I now have some work experience to draw upon when job-seeking—proof-reading newsprint, cataloguing library books, editing a weekly paper, and teaching aphasic children. And my speech is now understandable most of the time.

Surely something will turn up for me!

6

Journey Steps at Home

A t home, my most dreaded expectations are realized. Home *is* boring, and there's nothing to do. Mother is either out selling *My Bookhouse* or playing bridge. Dad is still teaching. My brother, David, is no longer home.

Dave is already following a varied career path. After his freshman year at Wesleyan University in New Haven, Connecticut, he spends a year as an interpreter for the U.S. Army in Japan. On his return, he spends two and a half more years at Wesleyan and graduates with high honors and Phi Beta Kappa in June 1949. There follow three years at Yale Law School. David is married to Frances, the sweetheart of his teen years, and now, in 1953, is working for a law firm in Philadelphia.

There is now little for me to do except read, write letters and

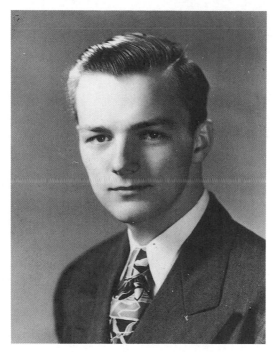

David Webb, age nineteen

watch Dad's pride and joy—a newly purchased television set. My only companion and constant lap cover is Ginger. Whenever I back up to my easy chair and prepare to sit down, my dog makes a flying leap and lands in my lap just as my bottom hits the chair. She then acts as my book holder until I command, "Ginger, get down!"

One afternoon not long after my return from the institute, Dad comes home from work and says excitedly, "Ruth, how would you like to volunteer at the Ardmore School for Retarded Children? It is run by the County Association for Retarded Children. I have just talked with the principal, Mr. Rizzo, and he is willing for you to observe the children and to write reports on them. He can't pay you any money, but it will be good experience for you. I will drive you to and from Ardmore on Monday, Wednesday, and Friday. Will you try it?"

I exclaim, "Oh yes! Thank-you, Dad! This is an opportunity to practice my training with aphasic children. Now I'll show old Professor Crusen that I can use my master's degree."

So I do volunteer observations in the small school from February to June, 1954. I attend the morning assembly and two classes of five to seven students. Each day I focus on one child and record his/her social behavior, length of task attention, and retention of curriculum material. That night at home I type a report for Mr. Rizzo.

One afternoon after school, a young man in a clerical collar and gray suit knocks at the door. He announces, "I am Joe Bishop, pastor of the Presbyterian Church. I understand you have just returned from Kansas and want to get acquainted with our community. Would you like to attend the Young Adult Group [YAG] at our church? They meet every Sunday night at 5:30 for supper and an evening program. I'm sure that they will be glad to pick you up."

I am excited and fairly shout my yes. Then I look at Mother. I sense she is trying to say yes, but wanting very much to say no. At this point, I do not understand why she is hesitating. Doesn't she want me to go?

She finally speaks. "Mr. Bishop, this is a wonderful opportunity for Ruth. I know she will enjoy getting out and meeting new friends. Are you sure she won't be imposing?"

I flush with embarrassment at Mother's question. Why does Mother think I will impose on the group?

Mr. Bishop winks at me. "Not at all. Ruth will be a great asset for the group. I will ask the membership committee to arrange her transportation."

For the next five years, I look forward to Sunday evening and the fellowship of thirty to forty young adults. After a community supper, there are always very interesting programs, which include lectures on art and current events, political debates, and musical recitals.

At these meetings, I get to know many people my age in the church and meet many good friends and acquaintances. The YAGs are all young professional people and are divided quite equally between married couples and single gals and guys. One result arising from my attendance at the YAGs meetings is that I learn to drink coffee. *Good* coffee remains a pleasure for me to this day.

One year I am asked to write a play for Easter, and so *The One Prized Lamb* appears. The main character of the play is Simon of Cyrene, the man commandeered by Roman soldiers to carry the cross of Jesus, along the way to Calvary. Through Simon's eyes and deeds, the play reports the crucifixion of the man called Christ.

When the cross is laid on Simon's shoulders, he seethes with anger. He curses God when his younger son, Rufus, reports that his elder son, Alexander, has mistakenly sacrificed the prized lamb that he, Simon, has been saving for the passover meal. His rage is now doubled and gushes out in violent torrents.

Simon's black mood turns to wonder and repentance as he witnesses the crucifixion. He now realizes that a much more "Prized Lamb" than his young ewe is being slain. When he hears the Roman centurion exclaim, "Surely this is the Son of God!" Simon sinks to his knees, saying, "This man is none other than our Messiah!"

My attendance at YAG intensifies the tension between Mother and me. Time and again we have royal battles centering around my need for emotional and social independence. It seems very difficult for her to let me go out without Dad or herself. I often try to understand Mother's reactions. I finally come to the conclusion that she simply cannot conquer her fear that she as well as I would be rejected by the community. She tries so hard to direct my activities that I begin to call her "Dear Tyrant," a name she does not relish. A very nervous person, she is constantly moving. Many times my slow movements greatly irritate her, and she lashes out at me.

A few examples: *Ruthie, why must you be so slow? Sit up straight. Speak plainly, Ruthie! Don't forget to go to the bathroom before getting in the car.* (This last reminder causes a tremendous battle between Mother and me, her 32-year-old daughter!) Mother makes great demands not only on me but also on herself, and she becomes so intent upon fulfilling those demands that she strikes out at anything or anyone who gets in the way of meeting her goals. However, Mother is determined to do everything she can to help me overcome my disability. In fact, she is the one who really starts and keeps me on my journey into personhood.

I become involved with the county United Cerebral Palsy (UCP) organization and get acquainted with Mildred and Robert Clayton. Mildred is the executive secretary and Robert is president of the board. We three seem to hit it off quite well. They invite me along on picnics, and Robert thinks nothing of carrying me considerable distances over rough ground. One evening, Mildred suggests that Robert invite me to be a member of the United Cerebral Palsy Board of Directors. He readily agrees, and thereafter I attend the monthly meetings.

There I meet Charles Alpine, a c.p. He is about my age and we share many interests—politics, chess, and UCP. He often stops to see me on his way home from his job. Sometimes we play chess.

During our games, I learn that Charles has a very hard time becoming independent from his mother. We spend many afternoons discussing this seemingly unsolvable problem.

Charles visits me at the Antlers, and we go for walks along the then quiet country roads, Charles on foot and I in my newly acquired electric chair. One afternoon I take him to the cemetery where Grandpa often took me in my wheelchair and where he and Nan now lie buried.

We climb a steep hill, and Charles pauses to catch his breath. He then steps in front of me, grabs my shoulders, kisses me, and says, "Ruth, I love you!"

At that propitious moment, the off-on switch on my chair begins to smoke. We hurry back to the Antlers in short stages, stopping every five minutes to let the switch cool.

Later that night when I am safe in bed, I agonize over this thought: Alas, my only chance for romance is ruined by an off-on switch. I was so afraid that Charles and I would be stuck in a graveyard with night approaching!

Although he never seeks another opportunity to kiss me, Charles visits me quite often and we remain good friends. One afternoon Charles suggests that we form a social group for c.p. adults. UCP will give us names of prospective members. And so the Adult C.P.'s of Delaware County is born.

The c.p. group eventually numbers ten persons, who have ten different stories to tell. These stories run the gamut of human misfortune. There are young people who are overprotected, neglected, alone, and angry. One is a husband and father, one is a homeowner, two have jobs, and the other six live with older parents. We become very close to each other as we share one another's problems. The fact that the group stays together for five years is evidence that it serves a real purpose.

At one of our meetings, Charles suggests that we present a panel discussion on problems of adults with c.p. to the board and to interested parents. This idea is adopted, and Charles and I agree to participate on the panel. Charles offers to talk about getting and holding a job. I opt to discuss parent-child relationships.

When it is my turn to speak, I begin, "Parents and their adult children with c.p. need to understand each other better. Young men and women try so hard to grow up, and parents sometimes work hard to keep them children. Parents are so used to taking care of their handicapped children that they don't realize that young people can make decisions for their own lives. We adult children want very much to grow up and to be independent."

I am very conscious of my speech and try extremely hard to pronounce every syllable correctly. Unfortunately, in my nervous effort to speak clearly, I lose my breath. Nevertheless, I feel that I am doing a good job in speaking. In fact, I am very proud of my performance.

Almost as soon as we get in the door at home, Mother attacks me for being out of breath. She says, "Ruth, why didn't you keep your voice pitched low when you spoke tonight? Your voice sounded terrible! I was so ashamed."

And I am crushed, so angry I cannot speak. As hot tears pour down my cheeks, I think, After I tried so hard to speak clearly, all Mother can do is to scold me.

Here again, Mother is voicing her great fear that I will not be accepted by the community at large because I am different. Display of my c.p. in public places—i.e., church, nursery school, YAG meetings, UCP board meetings, etc.—sharpens her fear that I, and perhaps she, will be rejected. Mother's outburst may have also been prompted by the subject of my talk.

There is always an underlying tension between Mother and me. I want to grow up and control my own life; she, perhaps without realizing it, fosters my dependence. A continual struggle ensues between us.

In September 1955, Maggie Machlin, director of the Swarthmore Presbyterian Nursery School, invites me to be a consultant. My task is to observe the children three mornings a week and write semi-annual reports for parents. She tells me later that God spoke to her one night and told her to hire me. So for three years, on Monday, Wednesday and Friday, I take my motor chair the three blocks to the church. I receive $15 a week and a lot of experience.

I observe the children during music and crafts periods and on the playground. The outdoor activities require me to be mobile, and so I use my big motor chair. Mother and Dad are reluctant to have me travel along the busy highway to the church. But I insist on going the three blocks to my job, even in the rain.

"What will people say?" Mother keeps asking.

At the nursery school, Maggie gives me freedom to experiment. I design a behavior rating scale to record each child's performance in daily activities. I then study drawings of the human figure by five-year-olds and give the Goodenough "Draw a Man" test to thirty-five youngsters. The results show that young children's figure drawings bear a close resemblance to their own appearance.

On one of the afternoons when we are riding in the car, Dad says, "Ruth, how would you like to have your own apartment on the first floor of our house? The screened-in porch can easily be converted to a bedroom and study for you, and the alcove off the fireplace will make a neat bathroom. I will put in a stall shower, toilet, and vanity to make your apartment complete."

I get very excited and exclaim, "Oh Dad, that will be wonderful! Then I won't have to climb the stairs, and you won't have to put in a banister on the last three steps. I won't have to bump down stairs on my rear."

"That's right," Dad smiles. "And Mommy won't have to worry about your falling downstairs."

I watch my apartment grow from a long side-porch to a bedroom and study, enclosed by knotty-pine paneling. My bedroom is separated from the study by ceiling-high bookcases on either side of a doorway leading from my room to the study. The French doors, which once opened onto the porch, now give me privacy from the rest of the house. Dad buys me a desk and a boudoir chair. I spend many hours at the desk and in my easy chair with my friend, Ginger.

To enable me to get outside independently, Dad puts in a door with an easy-to-turn knob and builds a small porch with a railing around it. A ramp with a forty-five-degree slope leads to the shed which houses my wheelchair. I am very elated when I can rise, shower, dress, and, after breakfast, open my own front door and walk down the ramp, unlatch the shed door, get in my chair, and drive off. I am now practically independent.

Ginger enjoys the apartment too. She is now in my lap most of the time. At night the little dog sleeps in the crook of my knees. When nature calls her, she jumps down and stands breathing in my face until I wake to let her out. Ginger never leaves the yard, except to try to follow me to church on the street behind our house.

My dog is a lifelong chum. She lives to be fifteen and a half years. On the night of her death, she walks away from the house, a very unusual act. The next morning a friend finds her dead on the highway two miles away. My grief is compounded with guilt, because

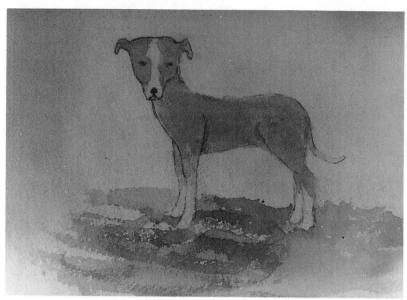

Ginger, painted by Kaye McKinnon

before letting her out, I scold her for messing the floor, something she hadn't done since her puppyhood. I still miss her. There will never be another Ginger.

It is August 1957, during a long, boring summer at the Antlers, that a letter comes from Nanette Butler of my Syracuse days. She tells me about Camps Farthest Out (more familiarly called CFO). These are interdenominational prayer camps which emphasize physical and inner healing in the name of Jesus Christ. Her mother-in-law, Carola Bell Williams, is a leader and will be at the CFO in Lima, New York. Nanette urges me to write the camp registrar and ask if she can find someone to assist me during camp. She ends her letter, "Ruth, I am sure you will find CFO a spiritually refreshing experience."

I write Ann Dunning, camp registrar, and in a week there is a reply to my letter: "Yes, there will be someone to help you. We are very happy that you are coming."

After an all-day drive, Dad and I arrive at the small college in

Lima. Ann Dunning greets me on the low porch of a college dorm and introduces Alice Menard, my helper.

After supper, our speaker, Glenn Clark, introduces Camps Farthest Out. He begins, "In 1930, when I was professor and athletic coach at Macalester College in St. Paul, God gave me a vision. He asked me to find a place where 'athletes of the spirit' could go farthest toward Him in body, mind and spirit. At my invitation, several spiritually gifted persons gathered for a two-week camp in North Carolina and began to pray continuously. Lo, miracles happened. Bodies, minds, and spirits were healed. That camp has spawned the present thirty-five camps, which are scattered all over the world. God is using CFO to show His love to the world."

After Glenn's talk, the evening proceeds with lively hymn singing and introductions to the week's activities. All programs are designed to relax body and mind so that spiritual creativity may flow freely in each camper. There are two talks each day. "Devotion in Motion" and "Creative Arts" (writing and music) occur after the morning message. In the late afternoon, prayer groups of six to twelve persons meet for an hour and a half.

Glenn teaches that there is a way to pray that opens the subconscious and allows the soul's sincere desire to express itself. He asserts, "Then prayers get answered!" He claims that prayer groups are the most important part of camp.

After the week's six sessions, prayer group members grow very close to one another and willingly share their problems. They then join hands and pray, sometimes laying hands on each other. In this atmosphere of love, miracles do happen. Interpersonal disputes dissolve, loved ones are healed, and even nonfunctioning arms are raised in praise and thanksgiving.

Besides prayer, Glenn's talks emphasize a here-and-now relationship with Jesus Christ. Grandpa's words, "He will always be with you," stir again in me. I am awed by the realization that I can actually communicate with Jesus and He will guide me.

The camp's "Devotion in Motion" program fascinates me. Carola

Williams leads this dancing to hymns. She is very tall, slim, and graceful and is a beautiful sight to watch when she is dancing in her white dress on the green grass. I sit in the middle of the dance circle and imitate her motions as best I can. She smiles and encourages me to continue worshiping with my arms. One of my favorite songs that she interprets is "The Lord Knows the Way through the Wilderness. All We Have to Do Is Follow."

On Wednesday afternoon, Carola and I sit under the big oak trees to talk about Nanette, her daughter-in-law and my fellow student at Syracuse University. Within ten minutes we feel as if we have known each other all our lives. It is an incredible experience!

Carola is not satisfied with the care Alice is giving me, so she pays Alice her week's wages and has her move out of my room. Then Carola moves in all her things and takes over my care. She confides to me later that she has a sister with c.p.

Carola becomes my close friend for forty-two years. For a year or so we write each other every week, and she frequently drives from Albany, New York, to pick me up for a three-day visit in her home. In spite of her leadership position, she takes care of me at camp for eight summers at Silver Bay, the well-known YMCA camp on Lake George, New York.

Many wonderful experiences of God's presence come to me at Silver Bay CFO. First of all, Carola's devoted attention makes me realize I am loved for who I *am*, not for what I am trying to do, i.e., get a job. This is a great revelation. Carola keeps saying to me, "Ruth dear, don't worry about *doing*, just *be*."

Carola's faith amazes me. She says, "Give your troubles to the Lord and He will take care of them." Through the years, she supports me many times with her optimistic faith. She strongly believes that the Lord brings good out of trouble.

Her play *The Supreme Court* illustrates her faith that God's forgiveness is available to all. It is the story of seven women who wake after a bus crash to find themselves in the Ultimate Supreme Court. When the play opens, the audience sees Carola sitting in one of seven empty chairs, each of which is draped with a different colored shawl. As Carola changes chairs, she becomes a different woman with a unique voice and body movements. In this way, the seven women come to life before the audience's very eyes.

Each of the seven women is angry and afraid because she has suffered unspeakable cruelty in the Holocaust, poverty and prostitution in city slums, or character-destroying abundance in wealthy homes.

The last character, a young blind girl, greatly impresses me. Instead of mourning her lot, she thanks God for her loving parents and friends as well as for the beauty she has known through taste, smell, and touch. Her faith in God is rewarded when she receives her sight, and she now sees the roses she has known through smell and touch.

As I ponder my life and my journey into personhood, I wonder if I will ever be able to thank God for my disability. Carola, by symbolizing God's love for me, helps me begin to thank Him for my life.

I am surprised and delighted by the accepting atmosphere of CFO. The camp meets each one where he or she is and motivates people to go "farthest out" toward God. Bathed in love, people open their arms and hearts to each other, and camp becomes one big love feast. Within three days I feel accepted and loved by the whole camp. Carola is the prime example of the love I find at CFO.

However, for some CFOers, this love is intoxicating and creates a desire to remedy the evils of the world. When these campers first meet me, they want to pray for my physical healing. At Lima, I am approached by an enthusiastic minister who, without asking me, gathers together five or six people to form a "healing circle" around me to pray for my healing. I am greatly embarrassed and totally reject the idea that I can be healed physically. Carola helps me understand this experience. "His intentions are good, Ruth," she says. "Try to see the love in them."

Many times I have felt at the mercy of these overenthusiastic healers. At these times, I am almost torn in two. I want healing so much, but I am terribly embarrassed to be the center of the circle. Then I wonder whence my healing is supposed to come, God or the human hands on my head.

Over the years, I learn to ask for inner healing from fear, anger, frustration, etc. One by one, great emotional blocks have melted and continue to do so. There are still many knots to be untied, but at least I know God is there when I am ready to seek His help in freeing my tangled shuttle.

Mother and I have several remarkable experiences with the Holy Spirit at CFOs through the years. One evening in the Silver Bay chapel, Tommy Tyson, a great evangelist from South Carolina, preaches about the Holy Spirit. Suddenly, a strong wind starts from the narthex and sweeps through the Norman-style church with a mighty Pentecostal surge. That night there is no doubt in any one's mind that we have been visited by the Holy Spirit.

The stone chapel, with its Norman arches, is the site of other remarkable experiences for me. There Tommy tells me that the Holy Spirit is within me. And it is there I saw a bright light around Dr. Frank Laubach, world literacy specialist, as he broke the Communion bread.

Through CFO, my lifelong anger about my c.p. and its attendant rejections, my helplessness, and loneliness begins to fade. God becomes real, and His presence is manifested many times to me. I experience immersion for renewed baptism in the Warwick swimming pool and receive the name Joy from that year's speaker, my pastor and friend, the Rev. Joe Bishop.

I return from camp resolving to study the Bible and meditate every day. Unfortunately, I never meditate as long as I should. Even so, God continues to bless me greatly for forty-two years through Camps Farthest Out. To me the CFO camps have been God's signposts on my journey into personhood.

I can hardly wait to return home to my friend Lynn Sterling, who is a mystic and spends much time praying. I infect her with my enthusiasm for CFO, and she suggests that we invite three other friends to join us in a prayer group. Our friends accept, and we meet weekly for reading, discussion, and prayer. A close bond of friendship and love quickly forms among us. We feel related to each other as we share our hopes and fears and pray for each other every day.

After twenty years of running the Antlers, my parents finally sell it to a young couple in May 1955, thus ending their long summers of labor. My parents and I quickly pack up and leave the big white inn, which holds memories of toilsome days and wonderful guests. I am very glad I won't have to spend any more boring summers at the Antlers.

Home again in Swarthmore, Mother and Dad immediately make plans to visit friends in California. They promise me to return in two weeks. My friend Mildred agrees to stay with me while her husband, Robert, is on a fishing trip. Two weeks pass quickly and then two more days. My parents do not return. Mildred reluctantly leaves to take care of the returning Robert.

I am alone for two more weeks. My parents have left no address or phone number so I cannot contact them. When I run out of groceries, my friend Dora shops for me, so I survive until their return.

When Mother and Dad return, I ask them why they stayed the extra two weeks. Mother gives a surprising answer: "We were having such a good time and our friends wanted us to stay, so we stayed!" Perhaps both my dear parents were simply burned out because of their many responsibilities, including taking care of me.

One morning a month later, Mother is making my bed. As she raises her arms to pull the blanket up, a sharp pain goes through her chest and she exclaims, "Ruth, I can't make your bed this morning. I have a very sharp pain in my chest." Mother's first angina attack puts her in the Valley Forge Army Hospital for eleven weeks. The sudden release from pressure of the Antlers seems to be too much for her.

Dad and I keep house, and he does his best to cook good meals for us. He likes steak, and so we eat that often for dinner. Soup and dry cereal are often on the menu. I tease Dad about graduating from the U.S. Army's Cooks and Bakers School. He answers jokingly, "I don't want to show you what I know. Then Mommy will have me cooking all the time!" He helps me with my buttons and bows, and twice a week we drive to Valley Forge Hospital to visit Mother.

Mother comes home after eleven weeks in the hospital and slowly regains her strength. At times she continues to have angina, and she keeps a nitroglycerine tablet handy. Several years later, Mother's angina disappears during a healing service at Warwick CFO. Her healing comes through the hands of Tommy Tyson. Never again does she have angina.

In spite of my experience with God's love at CFO and my busy schedule, I spend long and lonely days alone at home. Much of the time, I worry about my future: If I can't get a job what will become of me? Will I end up in an institution? Then I'll never get a chance to help people and become a worthwhile person. At this point, I begin to cry. Some days I cry for hours.

One afternoon Rev. Joe is walking by my door to his home, which is the third house from our corner. I am alone and feel very desperate. As he passes our house, Joe has a strong urge to come up my ramp, open the door, and walk into my apartment. He finds me in the bathroom weeping.

"Ruthie dear, whatever is the matter?" he exclaims as he wraps his arms around my shoulders.

"I'm just no good! I can't get a job. No one wants a c.p. I want to die!"

"Well, Ruthie [Joe always puts the *ie* on my name but I love him so much, I can't complain], I don't agree that you are no good. How about coming to my study tomorrow afternoon to talk about these problems which are troubling you so much. Perhaps with the Lord's help, we can find some answers."

Thereafter, I see Joe every week for counseling about my fear regarding my purpose in life. Joe helps me uncover my great anger with God about my disability and my feeling of rejection by society.

We also discuss my mother's reluctance to let me go out alone. Joe tries to assure me that her reaction is a normal one and that all mothers are afraid to let go of their children. "Your handicap makes it doubly hard for your mother to relinquish you to the wider community," he says.

Joe is very loving and concerned about my problems. During the three years of our sessions I grow very fond of him. He helps me gain a better understanding of Mother and Dad and encourages me to keep looking for the right job. "You will find your job someday when the Lord knows you are ready," Joe says.

One day in May 1954, I hear that Oral Roberts, the well-known television evangelist, is holding healing meetings in nearby Trenton, New Jersey. I wonder, Could he heal my c.p.? So I ask Joe to take me to one of Mr. Roberts's meetings, and he readily agrees.

The next Saturday morning, Joe and Carrie, his wife, pick me up for the drive to the Trenton fairgrounds, where the Oral Roberts Crusade tents are pitched. At the door of an enormous tent, an usher waves us to the right into the "invalid" tent. Here my eyes are dazzled by row upon row of people in wheelchairs and wheeled litters. I think, No wonder Jesus was touched by the suffering crowds.

At last the great man enters the tent and proceeds around the circles of "invalids." A very strong wind moves before him as he steps from one person to the next. When Oral Roberts reaches me, he stops and looks me straight in my eyes.

I think, Can you really heal me?

After looking at me a full minute, he exclaims loudly, "Be healed!" Giving me a terrific whack between my shoulders, he passes on. I sit there stunned for a moment. I don't feel anything in me has changed. Yet I want to be sure.

I look at Joe standing in front of me. "I want to see if I can walk," I murmur. Without a word, Joe raises the footboards on my chair and pulls me up to stand. I step off with Lefty, but to my deep disappointment, Righty drags behind as it always has. And I am still very much afraid of standing alone in space. Crestfallen beyond words, I say to Joe, "Let's go home."

After this experience, I am very depressed for several months. What good am I if even God won't heal me? I think it again and again.

During these days, Joe often visits our home and chats with my parents. He tries hard to allay Mother's worries about me and to make her understand that my refusal to let her guide me in little things is quite normal for an adult my age.

"Yes," says my mother, "but how will Ruth manage when Billy and I are gone?"

My pastor later tells me that he answers my worried mother by saying, "Many parents ask me that question. Most children find their own answer. I think Ruthie will surely find her own solution to this problem, with God's help."

Then my beloved minister concludes his reminiscences about my dear mother. "Ruthie," he says, "you and your mother were so close that you often stumbled over each other."

One evening in January 1956, Joe raps at my door. As he enters, I know what he is going to say. "Ruth," he begins, "I have answered a call to a church in Boston. This is a great opportunity for me because I will be able to take courses with the great theologian, Paul Tillich. I will be his assistant so I will be in daily contact with him. I will miss this church and I will miss you, but I cannot turn down this opportunity."

"When will you leave?" I ask trembling.

"June fifteenth," he replies. "I have five months to finish my job here. You and I will have lots of talks in that time."

I am devastated. I actually ache as I begin to say good-by to Joe. I hurt every time I pass a church, and this continues for six months. I cannot imagine that Joe will remain my friend throughout life.

In February, Agnes Sanford, a well-known author and healer in the Episcopal Church, gives an evening talk at my church. I invite Carola to come down from Albany. Lynn and Mildred also are present. Of course, Mother and Dad attend.

At a previous meeting, I had asked Mrs. Sanford if she could heal me. She forthrightly declared that it was beyond her power to heal cerebral palsy.

Dad, not knowing of that meeting, asks Mrs. Sanford to come and see me after her talk. As she approaches, I suddenly become two persons, an actor and an observer. The observer is horrified at what the actor is doing but is powerless to stop her. The unruly actor part of me is shouting, "No, no! Don't come!"

Mrs. Sanford stops uncertainly. My parents stand transfixed on either side of me. The few people still in the church look at me in astonishment, and everyone is motionless. I sense that Joe has left the church.

And then out of the corner of my left eye, I see Joe Bishop coming up the aisle to my pew. I burst out crying. When he reaches me, Joe whispers softly. "Don't cry now, Ruth, wait until later. I think what you really want is to talk to Mrs. Sanford alone."

I gasp, "Will you be there?"

Joe nods and tells my parents he will bring me home. Then he goes to find Agnes. Finally he escorts me into his study to meet her. Agnes stands near a window and begins to speak. "There were years I couldn't go near a window without wanting to jump. The Lord cured me of this desire. Now, I don't have enough faith to heal cerebral palsy—I'm only a little engine and can't pull a big train—but the Lord has given me power to heal your impulse for suicide!"

Joe and I look at each other in amazement, and he tells Agnes, "Yesterday Ruth told me she wants to end her life."

Agnes nods knowingly. "Do you want me to pray for you?" she asks me.

I whisper, "Yes."

While Joe kneels, Agnes puts her hands on my head and prays. I feel as if a cup of warm soup is being poured into the top of my head. Warmth flows through my neck, my chest, my legs, throughout my whole being. For ten or more days, I feel as light as a feather floating on air. The self-destructive urge does not trouble me again for two years.

The next morning, Joe and I review the previous night's events. Joe's experience was even more amazing than my own. After Agnes's talk, he slipped across the snow-covered road to his study and sat down at his desk to work on his next sermon. He had just put pen to paper when he felt an irresistible urge to return to the church. In a trance, he dashed across the street and into the church.

Still not knowing what to do, my bewildered pastor started down the three-hundred-foot aisle and saw me. He tells me, "Then my mission became clear. I was to take you to Agnes."

"How did you know what to say to stop my crying?" I ask.

Joe answers tenderly, "I don't know, Ruthie. We were all in God's hands last night." Then he adds, "Our experience shows me that healing comes in God's time and in the way He designs. We initiated the rather unfortunate meeting with Oral Roberts, and it didn't turn out so well. Last night's events were entirely orchestrated by the Lord, and all of us were touched."

Carola, Lynn, and Mildred are very elated at the manifestation of God's grace. I feel that the presence of my friends at this event confirms the fact that we had a great encounter with God.

For me, the healing session with Agnes Sanford and Joe is a deeply redeeming experience. Even after forty years, recalling that wonderful night in February 1955 sends an awesome thrill up my spine. Although circumstances may make me momentarily forget this life-changing meeting with the Lord, I will always remember that memorable night when God, the Great Spirit, shows me in no uncertain terms that He is directing my journey into personhood.

7

On the Ph.D. Trail

One bright October morning in the fall of 1958 Dad says to me, "Pilikia, let's look for a university where you can get an advanced degree. What about you, Mother, and I taking a trip to visit some graduate schools?"

So within the week the family sets out upon a delightful journey through the brightly colored foliage of New England and the Midwest. At Boston University, the chairperson of the Psychology Department accepts me but alas, there are no barrier-free dormitories. We then visit the University of Michigan in Ann Arbor and Michigan State University in Lansing. Both schools accept me—quite a switch from being rejected by three graduate schools after graduating from Drew. I make no commitment to either university but decide to wait until I see the famous program for disabled students at the University of Illinois.

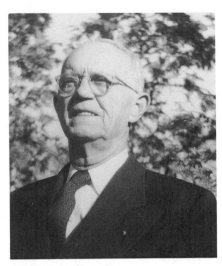

William Webb, 1960

In the education building on the UI campus, we meet the coordinator of graduate studies, Dr. Wade, who describes the Ph.D. program in education and outlines the courses and examinations that I will have to take. When he cautiously suggests that I consider an associate doctor's program which will take only two years and will not involve language exams, I decline by declaring, "I want a Ph.D.! It's all or nothing." The UI is my choice of the four universities we visit because it has a rehabilitation program for disabled students.

This program is headed by the quixotic and peripatetic Matthew Maloy. Matt, as he is called, looks at me and my disability very skeptically and declares that he doubts the veracity of my transcript from Drew. He acts as if I am too dependent on others to be in graduate school. When we leave his office, my indignant mother tells me never to consult him about my problems. I never do.

I enter the university when the second term begins in February 1959 and attend the first meeting of the Disabled Students Organization. I soon learn that Matt is bombastic and excitable. To make his students become self-reliant, he exhorts us to be aggressively independent and not ask favors from anyone. I react quite negatively to this all-or-nothing attitude. Everybody needs help sometime. However, by the end of my first term, my disagreement with Matt is not as strong. After all, he has enabled me and many other disabled students to join the academic, sports, and social life of the campus.

The rehab program has buses to take disabled students around campus. These buses circle the campus every hour, transporting students from dorms to class buildings, the library, and the gym, and then back again.

Although my new, more compact electric chair goes only three miles an hour, it brings me more freedom than I have ever had. I am thrilled the first time I descend on the bus lift to the cement walk leading two hundred feet to the library entrance. Because Matt has insisted that every building be ramped, I can actually go from building to building by myself and even shop in the surrounding town. I feel very independent.

It doesn't take long to meet my advisor. Professor Walter Hiland, affectionately called Dr. Walt by all his students, is professor of vocational rehabilitation. He is a prince of a guy and a very thorough lecturer. To me he is very kind and is always ready to listen to my problems. He sympathizes with my anxieties about my job placement and never ignores the problems created by my cerebral palsy.

Dr. W. E. Newmarket, Dr. Walt's associate, is a big, hearty, joking guy. I enjoy his course, "Psychology of the Handicapped." He maintains that there is no special psychology of the handicapped. Disabled people respond to the stress of being different by employing healthy as well as unhealthy adaptations, just as everybody else does.

Dr. Newmarket firmly believes that my disability prevents me from administering psychological tests, and he will not permit me to take his course in individual intelligence testing. I persuade him to give me an individual study course in which ten students are rated according to the Wechsler Adult Intelligence Scale by a handicapped examiner (me) and an able-bodied student. Of course, the able-bodied student obtains the best results as judged by Dr. Newmarket, but my report on the project is accepted by the dean in lieu of a master's thesis.

During my first month at UI, my physical endurance is severely taxed. All day long, I suffer from thirst and fatigue. Two and three classes on alternate days, meeting buses on time, getting to meals, studying, dressing and bathing—all this stretches me to the point of exhaustion. I am completely independent in routine self-care and have help from Connie, a pleasant sophomore, only in doing laundry and in caring for my nails. In spite of Mother's objection, I cut my hair short to avoid having to set it every night.

My first term I room with a nineteen-year-old sophomore whose major objective is to have a good time. Her constant phone conversations annoy me greatly when I am trying to study, so after my first semester, I move to another dorm where I have my own room for the next four years. At my request, the university carpenter makes a stool which can be firmly wedged between the wall and the tub in the dorm bathroom so I can take my own baths whenever my study schedule permits. I am delighted with this added independence.

Among the many rehab students, Bob Linch stands out. He has very severe cerebral palsy and is president of the Disabled Students' Organization. He takes a liking to me and introduces me to the problems and joys of campus life.

Bob has been raised to try everything that comes his way and to relate to the nonhandicapped majority by charming those around him with his wit and good humor. He engages in all the social activities of dorm life and readily joins the boys' drinking bouts. He is a great flirt and has many "conquests" under his belt. Bob invites adventure in spite of his very poor speech and complete lack of hand control (he cannot feed or dress himself).

This colorful guy sets out to educate me in the good times of campus life. Many afternoons I take coffee breaks with Bob at the union cafeteria and enjoy wide-ranging conversations. Little do I realize that this amazing man will play an important role in my finding a job.

Perhaps my most intellectual friend on campus is Wilga Rivers, who is from Australia. We meet in my second UI term in three different classes. Wilga is very effusive and energetic, and we immediately become friends. She is blessed with an extremely high energy level and can work twelve hours without ceasing and then go for dinner and a show. Wilga is an untiring conversationalist and can lead an interesting discourse on any subject. Our almost-weekly outings to plays, operas, and concerts give me many educational experiences I would not have had without her.

During my third year at UI, I become so depressed that I ask for help at the Student Counseling Center. I am worried about finding a job, and Rev. Joe's departure still haunts me. I am assigned to Dr. John Henning, professor of psychology, a kind, middle-aged man. He works with me during my last two terms.

The critical incident in these counseling sessions is the discovery of an old mental wound or neurotic core, which stems from being stripped in front of clinic doctors at NEIL, my first boarding school. Dr. Henning leaves me with at least one less piece of emotional baggage.

My third summer at UI is the season for my first comprehensive examination. I spend five weeks at home trying desperately to review all the notes from eighteen courses taken over three years. When I return to campus, my friend Peggy, a junior in the church Sunday evening fellowship, offers to take my dictation of the exam questions. Her kind suggestion decreases my anxiety and again seems to be a providential signpost upon my path. I am relieved when the two exam days are over. When Dr. Walt calls me at home four days later to tell me I passed my first comp, I breathe a great big sigh of relief.

In September 1961, Dr. Walt begins his counseling practicum by saying, "To become good counselors, you must develop a therapeutic personality. This course will give you many opportunities to develop such a personality."

Little do I realize the form the development of my therapeutic personality will take. I do my practice counseling at the nearby U.S. air base. Sergeant Martin, the man in charge of the counseling center, is very reluctant to give me any clients. Week after week, every Wednesday and Friday afternoon from one to four o'clock, this man lets me sit in a small room and do nothing. One day he even suggests that I not come to the base at all. When I tell Dr. Walt, he shrugs his shoulders and says, "Ruth, all behavior has a cause. Someday, perhaps, you will cause the Sgt. Martins of this world to change their behavior toward disabled counselors."

My opportunity to help Sgt. Martin change his attitude and therefore his behavior toward the handicapped comes on the last Friday afternoon of the term, when only two of us student counselors show up. The other student has a client as soon as he arrives. A very worried-looking airman now enters and asks for help. Sgt. Martin looks around and sees no counselor but me. He sighs and leads the man into my room. I quickly turn on the tape recorder and say, "Tell me what is troubling you."

The airman rambles on for an hour while I listen and try to reflect his feelings. I gather that he is very disturbed about being disciplined for coming in after curfew. This is just the beginning of a long list of grievances against his sergeant in particular and the Air Force in general.

When reviewing the session tape with me, Dr. Walt comments that my only mistake is that as a new counselor, I interpret the client's words too often rather than reflecting his feelings.

After giving me an A— for the practicum with U.S. airmen, Dr. Walt suggests that my internship be taken at the Student Rehabilitation Center on campus. I hesitate because I know my old disbeliever, Matt Maloy, has never quite overcome his aversion to me and will not make my internship at the rehab center very profitable.

As a counseling intern, I am supposed to attend the center's weekly staff meetings. Matt tries to prevent my attendance at these meetings by not offering me a ride to the site of the meetings.

When Dr. Walt hears of my problem, he insists that Matt include me in the staff deliberations. Thereafter, I am present for the weekly meetings, but Matt still refuses to give me any clients to counsel. This semester, instead of the three wasted afternoons of my internship, I am idle only one afternoon a week. Matt's excuse is that his director of counseling is ill and is unable to supervise me. Dr. Walt is well aware of the situation and gives me an A − for the course. I'm not sure how much therapeutic ability I develop in these two counseling courses, but my patience is certainly exercised. In my third year at UI, I begin searching for a subject for my dissertation. I spend many wakeful nights trying to fit bits and pieces of thoughts together. I know I want to learn more about how attitudes toward disabled people are formed. In July 1961, I attended a meeting for adults with c.p. held by the Philadelphia United Cerebral Palsy. The sights and sounds of a hundred c.p.'s in a small lecture room are traumatic and unforgettable.

I begin to wonder how abnormal speech, appearance, and movement influence formation of discriminatory attitudes toward disabled persons. I ask myself, Are there any theories of perception to support this idea? It takes me a year in the library to find and summarize 250 articles and papers on theories of perception and attitude formation.

The three questions finally posed by my proposal are these:

1. Does the way in which a person organizes visual perception influence discriminatory attitudes toward the physically handicapped?

Procedure: Identify perceivers who see their surroundings as wholes and those who see them as parts with Witkins' Perception Test.

2. Which of these three observable aspects of physical handicap—abnormal speech, appearance, or movements—is the most

important factor in forming adverse attitudes toward the physically disabled?

Procedures: A. Design a "social distance scale" to separate the influence of abnormal speech, appearance, and movements on the perception of nondisabled observers. B. Confirm discriminatory attitudes toward disabled students by administering Yukor's "Attitudes Toward the Handicapped Scale."

3. Which are more influential in forming attitudes toward the disabled, styles of perceiving or levels of familiarity?

Procedure: Determine the effect of familiarity by comparing group means on the "Attitudes Toward the Handicapped Scale" to see whether strangers, classmates, and roommates attain group acceptance scores in ascending order. The relationship between perceptual styles and the level of familiarity with disabled students will then be correlated to ascertain the relationship between acceptance scores and perceptual styles.

I present this proposal to my committee, and with their approval, I round up three groups of twelve first-year students who are roommates, classmates, and strangers in regard to disabled students.

My test results lead to three conclusions:

1. Perceptual styles, i.e., tendencies to see one's surroundings as wholes or as separate parts, have little effect on social acceptance of physically disabled students.

2. Negative attitudes toward the disabled are confirmed by Yukor's scale; abnormal speech is the disabling characteristic which is the most annoying to able-bodied students.

3. Roommates, the subjects most familiar with disabled students, are more accepting than classmates, and classmates are more accepting than strangers. This supports my hypothesis that levels of familiarity influence attitudes toward physically handicapped students more than do perceptual styles.

At Easter 1963, I spend three weeks at home dictating the first five of eight chapters of my dissertation to Mother. While typing my thesis, my dear secretary-mother suggests that she is entitled to a corner of my Ph.D. I tuck her wish away for future reference. I return to UI on a Sunday evening, just three weeks before my final comprehensive exam. This intervening time proves to be fraught with frustrations.

My trouble begins with the cab driver who brings me to the dorm from the airport. On arriving at the front door, I ask the man, "Where's my briefcase?" The bag holds all my library notes and the thesis copy just finished by the professional typist.

The man stammers, "I . . . I think the other taxi driver took it. I will call him right away and have him bring it."

My heart sinks and I say to the man, "You will get your money when I get my briefcase!" This declaration is a very unusual utterance for me. Most of the time when I am frightened, I cannot speak. It is an agonizing half hour before the second cab arrives and delivers my briefcase. By that time I am in tears.

The next morning another problem presents itself. I am dismayed to hear that my Canadian friend and the three student helpers recruited by the Employment Office are now in the throes of final exams and have no time to type for me.

In desperation, I phone Jenn Percy, a friend in need if ever there is one. Jenn, a doctoral candidate in special education, has attended classes with me. Having completed her work for the term, she devotes the next two weeks to typing the last three chapters of my dissertation as I dictate them.

Jenn also does much legwork for me by taking the first copies of my thesis to the local scribe and then delivering them to my committee members and to the graduate office.

I could never have finished without Jenn's help, yet she refuses any financial compensation. I often think that this dear friend's availability and willingness to help is a most propitious signpost proclaiming God's approval of this stage of my journey.

A week before commencement, I set out with my thesis to confer with Mrs. Brown, the official university dissertation typist, in her wheelchair-accessible shed. We discuss the hard and fast rules which the Graduate Office has for dissertation format. Our conversation is finished in half an hour.

Mrs. Brown then calls the rehab center to ask the bus driver to come for me. I start to go to the curb, which is about two hundred yards from the shed, when Rob, our driver, appears, stops, looks at me, and then moves on. I wait on the curb for an hour. A rainstorm comes and I get soaked to the skin before my slow chair reaches the shed. When the rain lets up four hours later, I am so angry I am crying. Rob finally comes back and picks me up. He gives no explanation and makes no apology for leaving me. I am a nervous wreck when I get back to the dorm, too late for lunch.

I have two other unpleasant experiences with bus drivers who seem not to like to wait for my slow chair. Or is it the appearance of my facial grimaces, the sound of my garbled speech, and the sight of my awkward movements? Or just my refusal to allow them to talk down to me? I console myself by remembering kind and good-natured Barney, the transportation director. Somehow there are always understanding persons to counteract the deeds of uncaring human beings.

My final comprehensive exam is scheduled on Saturday, two weeks before commencement. On Thursday before the fateful day, Mother calls to tell me that Dad is in the hospital with a blood clot in his left leg. He was mowing the yard when a terrible pain hit his leg. Mother found him groaning in agony when she came home two hours later. Mother indicates that the doctors are not very hopeful about Dad's recovery. If his condition improves, his leg will have to be amputated. I know he will not like that.

Even though I am worried sick about Dad, my dissertation has to be defended before the committee. The day finally comes, and I am very nervous and anxious as I wait in the office for the committee's summons. After what seems to be an interminable time, Dr. Walt comes to escort me into the conference room. Noticing my grim face, he puts his finger to his lips and encourages me to smile.

The committee members are seated around a long table. Dr. Walt

takes his place and motions me to sit beside him. He then announces, "The committee has decided to approve your dissertation
providing you rewrite your results less positively. We don't think the
statistical results provide absolute proof that familiarity factors are
more influential than perceptual styles in the formation of discriminatory attitudes. You will have to make these changes before your
degree will be awarded."

At this point, Professor Newmarket demands, "Why didn't you
change the variance of the test scores into standard deviations as I
asked? You know I'm trying to have all researchers use standard
deviation instead of variance." Dr. Newmarket turns red; he gets
up and walks out of the room in a great huff. I never see him again.

In my struggle to meet the committee's deadline, I have forgotten
to tell my data analyzers to turn the variance for the tests into
standard deviation intervals. The variance indicates how group
scores are placed about the mean. Standard deviation (SD) is the
square root of the variance.

Fortunately for me, the other committee members prevail, and in
a final vote, they declare that I pass this final comprehensive examination and the last hurdle for my Ph.D.

But how will I make the required changes in the weeks remaining
before commencement? On my way out of the conference room,
Dr. Walt leans over me and whispers, "Don't worry, Ruth. I will
make the changes for you."

"What about changing the variance into SD?" I ask. "All my ta-
bles will have to be retyped."

Dr. Walt hesitates a moment. Then he says softly, "Forget it."
And so my dear major prof makes all the changes recommended by
the committee. This is an almost unheard of favor.

Barney is waiting for me at the door of the counseling building
and is the first to greet me with the words, "Hi, Doc!" I feel exhausted as I lean against the bus door while the lift rises, and I
wearily say, "Thank you!"

Upon reaching my room, I call Dad's hospital and try to reach him. He is too ill to talk to me, but the nurse reports that he smiles triumphantly when he hears that I have passed my last comp.

The doctor now comes on the phone and, in answer to my inquiry about Dad's condition, gravely tells me that a second blood clot has formed in his intestines. In this year of 1963, there are no drugs to dissolve life-threatening blood clots. My poor dad has been suffering terribly for two weeks and dies in considerable pain on the evening of the day I pass my comp, June 2, 1963.

It is a bittersweet day. I achieve a long-sought, hard-earned goal but lose my dear dad in the same twenty-four hours. However, I sense his presence, and he seems to comfort and assure me that he is at peace.

Mother persuades me not to come home for the funeral. "Ruthie, your dad would want you to finish your work and get your Ph.D.," she says in a phone call. Rev. Joe and Carola both call to convey their sympathy. Joe also urges me to stay and get my degree. Although my heart wants very much to be present at the church service at home, I cannot possibly fly home for the funeral and turn in my dissertation on time. I have to stay and finish.

The following Wednesday afternoon at the same hour that my home church is having a funeral for Dad, the Rev. Durk of McGregor Church on campus holds a memorial service for him. Five of my friends attend the chapel service.

The days between comps and commencement pass very quickly until only one week remains. The Monday before commencement, Jenn and I drive up to White Horse, Wisconsin, for a job interview. There my c.p. friend, Bob Linch, has been a counselor at the Hebrew Career Center, a workshop and placement agency serving disabled people, for two years. He is now a supervisor, and in this capacity, he offers me a job as a beginning counselor.

Bob greets me warmly and says, "Ruth, we have an opening for a counselor to prepare clients for unskilled jobs. In your capacity as rehab counselor, you will also do adjustment counseling and interest surveying. When you think your clients are ready for jobs, our placement department will take over and find the kind of job you recommend for your client.

"You will work with a variety of disabled people—physically handicapped, emotionally disturbed, and perhaps some young delinquents. Will you accept a position as intern counselor at the beginning salary of six hundred dollars a month?"

I think for a moment and try to catch my breath. This is my first and only job offer and I must accept it, but Mother needs me at home for a little while. "Bob," I say, "I accept your offer. It will be fun to work here. The job really excites me, but I must stay at home with Mother for a few weeks to help her get over Dad's death."

"All right," says Bob. "We will expect you on the job four weeks from next Monday. In the meantime, I will try to find you a place to live."

My last week at the university passes with the speed of a fast express train. I am so tired and worn out from my all-out effort to finish my thesis. My weight is now eighty-four pounds. I need a physical examination to be sure that I can take on my new job.

I call the dean of women and ask her to recommend a physician. She gives me the name and phone number of a doctor whose office is on the north edge of campus. I phone immediately to schedule an appointment on Wednesday, the following afternoon.

After I wait for forty-five minutes, a nurse conducts me into a small room and asks what my problem is. "I need a physical exam," I explain. "I have been working very hard to finish my dissertation. I want to be sure I'm okay before accepting a job."

"A physical?" the nurse exclaims doubtfully. "I'll have to talk to the doctor about that. You are not his regular patient, so I don't think he will give you one."

She then goes out of the room and leaves me alone for twenty minutes. When she returns, she says, "The doctor does not see cripples. He suggests you go elsewhere."

I am very indignant and embarrassed. When I wheel out to the secretary's desk, she says, "Two dollars, please."

"For what?" I say, flushing with anger. I push the joystick on my chair very far ahead and shoot out the door without paying a cent. That day I learn that not all doctors adhere to the Hippocratic oath.

The dean is amazed by my reception at the doctor's office and makes an appointment for me with a woman physician on the staff of the university health center. I finally get a thorough exam, which assures me that I am ready to be a rehabilitation counselor.

Mother's plane lands at two o'clock Friday afternoon, the day before commencement. Jenn, my spirit guide in these last two weeks, and I drive to the airport to meet her. I will never forget how small and fragile Mother looks as she comes down the plane stairs. She is nearly bowed doubled with grief. She wraps her arms around me, begins to cry, and kisses me again and again. On our drive to the dorm, Mother tries hard to dry her tears while I tell her about my troubles in completing my dissertation.

When we get back to my room, I present Mother with a newly bound copy of my thesis. The first thing her eyes light upon is the side cover, where the second *b* in my last name is omitted. Of course, Mother insists that the volumes be rebound that very afternoon before they are finally presented to my committee. The trials and tribulations encountered in earning a Ph.D. are both great and small.

That evening Jenn and Connie take Mother and me to dinner at the University Tea House. We have a delicious steak dinner and spirited conversation about the joys and woes of the academic life. After dessert I give Mother a card bearing the letters Ph.D., embossed in gold. Attached to the bottom corner of the letter *D* is a silver pin. I say, "Mother, here is your corner of my Ph.D.!"

Commencement 1963 is the first event held in the university's new mushroom-shaped auditorium, which holds ten thousand people. It is an unforgettable moment when it is my turn to go up and be hooded. As I proceed slowly down the aisle in my motor chair, I feel very strongly that Dad is with me and that he is very happy. In my mind I hear him say, "Pilikia, you've made it. You are now a Ph.D.!"

As the dean puts the orange and blue hood over my head, images from the past four-and-a-half years flow rapidly through my mind. They are reminiscent of my struggles for physical and emotional independence as well as for mental and spiritual growth. Despite many frustrating moments, I have just passed a very significant signpost pointing to the future way of my journey. The certificate in my hand attests to the support of God-given friends and family in this final attainment of my long-coveted Ph.D.—my passport to a self-supporting job in a helping profession.

8

Struggles on the Career Path

"Miss, which will you have, toast or pancakes?"

A stoutish lady who seems to smile too brightly slaps the menu down before me. Feeling denied the chance to make my own decision, I reply, "Neither! I want one medium boiled egg and bacon, please." The woman looks at me suspiciously and then shouts my order into the kitchen.

While I eat my breakfast, I think of the fast and furious events of the past few days. It is my sixth week at home with Mother, who is barely recovering from Dad's death. She is wan and tired and very thin. She has not yet found words to express her grief, but I know she desperately wants me to stay with her a little while longer.

Thursday morning the telephone rings and Bob Linch, my counselor friend in Wisconsin declares, "Ruth, if you want the job, you'd better get out here!" This time Bob's irregular speech is clear and distinct.

"If you must go, you must, Ruthie," Mother declares from the living room telephone. "Don't lose your first real job because of me."

Bob continues, "We have persuaded the YMCA to give you a room. They are very reluctant to have a handicapped person live there, and it took much talking to get them to try you."

"I'll come out by TWA next Sunday afternoon," I say. "Can I take a cab to the Y?"

"No, Maurey Pohlson from the Hebrew Career Center will meet your plane and take you to the Y in White Horse. Then he'll pick you up Monday morning at 8:00 sharp. Have a good trip!" Bob signs off.

My daydream in the restaurant is interrupted by the waiter. "Now I suppose you want me to let you out of the shop."

I smile, "Please."

She opens the door, mumbling, "I don't mind doing little favors once in a while, but I won't do this every day!"

While I wait for my ride, I again lose myself in my memory. I think of my conversation with Mother as she packs my clothes, finally beginning to talk about Dad. "Ruth, your dad and I have looked forward to this day. He wanted you to realize your dream of supporting yourself. He always wished for a job which would give him prestige in his own eyes, and he never obtained a position that satisfied this desire. You are the one who will fulfill your dad's deep yearning for a meaningful job. I will miss you, but I want you to succeed. You have done very well so far to overcome your handicap. I'm sure you will do well in this new venture."

On the first Sunday of July 1963, Mother drives me to the airport and we tearfully say good-by at my plane's gate. In Chicago as I wait in my seat for the plane to take off, who should walk through the door and down the aisle but the CFO leader and my great friend, Tommy Tyson! When I tell him about my new job, he declares, "God's hand is in this new adventure. He is truly leading you." I then feel that our meeting is a signpost that God will bless my first job.

Maury Pohlson, who meets me at the airport, comes through the heavy, front doors and says cheerily, "Hello, are you ready to go to the Hebrew Career Center? We call it HCC for short. On the way, I will show you downtown White Horse."

We speed through ten blocks of tall office buildings and come quickly to the warehouse district. Maury eases his car into the parking lot, and we enter a wide, bare vestibule. A huge elevator takes us to the second floor.

There my friend Bob Linch meets me, and pushing his chair backward with his feet, he conducts me to my office at the end of a narrow, whitewashed hall. He opens the last door on the right and then wheels aside to watch my reaction. Inside are a desk, a bookcase, a filing cabinet, and one straight chair. There is just enough room for my motor chair to turn around.

"Your office is small but large enough for you to counsel one client at a time," Bob says. "To begin with, you have fifteen clients to get ready for placement. They include three emotionally disturbed patients, nine mentally retarded, and three physically handi‧ capped. There are staff and city directories near the phone. If you have any problems or need anything, call me." Saying this, Bob backs out the door and leaves me to prepare my schedule.

The first week passes fast. I meet my clients and become acquainted with their problems and potentialities for job placement. Mr. Randall, the placement officer, teaches me about the difficulties of finding jobs for disabled people. I am also assigned to supervise a section of the workshop which has thirty-five mentally retarded and emotionally disturbed clients.

Two young men, Bill and John, direct the hour-to-hour operation and keep me informed as to how many items are produced in a week. HCC signs subcontracts from local industries and assigns them to the section supervisors to complete. I enjoy going into my workshop section and watching the activity. Bill, John, and I hold

weekly meetings to discuss methods of improving the work adjustment of our clients. The job performance of each client is graded
daily, as is attendance, promptness, and ability to follow directions,
to finish a job, to maintain quality of work, and to sustain the
prescribed rate of output. Good relationships with supervisors and
peers are also a part of good work adjustment. Ratings on these
factors determine how near a client is to placement in the worka-
day world.

My supervisor, Mr. Blumegardner, is very understanding. I feel
free to go to him at any time, and he is always very helpful in
suggesting ways to overcome problems. He lets me make my own
mistakes and helps me in trying to compensate for them.

My most interesting client is Leanette Foster, a thirty-five-year-
old woman with cerebral palsy. She is a warm, friendly person who
is very depressed because she cannot get a job as a librarian, the
profession in which she is trained. Leanette has a peculiar walking
gait. As she puts her right foot forward, she turns her head to the
left side. This pattern is reversed when she steps with her left foot.
She then turns her head to the right.

I consult Dr. Bruce McCallister, the workshop's optometrist,
about Leanette's unusual walking pattern. Dr. McCallister comes
up with a surprising answer. He maintains that Leanette uses only
one eye at a time because the other eye is blocking its partner's
vision. Dr. McCallister thinks that this problem is caused by the
way Leanette holds her head. In order for her to see with her right
eye, she has to cock her head to the left. When she uses her left eye,
the position of her head blocks the vision of her right eye. In
Dr. McCallister's opinion, this situation cannot be improved because of Leanette's movement pattern.

Leanette's case makes me very interested in Dr. McCallister's
theory that the senses of sight, hearing, taste, and smell are closely
tied up with a person's movement patterns. I do not know now that
this perceptual motor theory will be the theoretical basis of my
work with profoundly retarded children.

Leanette and I work for many months on gaining a better emotional adjustment. We explore other job areas, such as filing, hostessing, proofreading, and so forth. Nevertheless, Leanette persists in sticking to her original goal of working in a library. Finally, Mr. Randall locates a part-time job for her as a reference person in a small library in Madison. A report six months later says that Leanette is living in a small apartment and her employer is satisfied with her work. This gives me immense fulfillment, and through the years, I am often inspired by Leanette's determination to carve out her own career.

After six months, HCC gives me supervisory responsibility. One day Mr. Blumegardner brings a good-looking, African American girl to my office and introduces her. "Dr. Webb, this is Miss Doreen Page, a beginning counselor. Give Doreen six of your clients and help her prepare them for job placement."

Then turning to Doreen, Mr. Blumegardner says, "Miss Page, feel free to come to Dr. Webb with any counseling problem."

Doreen is very forthright as she greets me, her new supervisor. "I will question you every step of the way," she asserts defiantly.

I think to myself, Doreen, you and I are going to have fun! And so a struggle for control begins. Doreen cannot take criticism from me, her white supervisor, and will not admit that she makes mistakes.

Mr. Blumegardner helps me take an objective view of my supervisee. "Let her make her own mistakes," he advises. "You can only help as much as she will let you."

While Doreen's resentment of me hurts, I understand her behavior. As a member of a social minority group, she has been discriminated against and excluded. I understand her anger because, after all, I, too, belong to a minority.

Meanwhile, things are not going well at the Y. The director, Mr. Hausmeister, does nothing to make my daily life easy. When I engage a waitress to do my laundry, he declares, "My waitresses are not paid to do laundry. The Y is not a social service agency!" When he catches me requesting help to open doors to the coffee shop, Mr. Hausmeister tells me that I am asking too many favors.

As soon as Bob hears about my troubles at the Y, he and his wife have dinner with me that night. Afterward he chides me for not tipping the waitresses enough for taking my tray through the cafeteria line. I sigh and remember Mother's persistent warnings to save my money. This is just one more bone of contention in my life at the Y. I am very angry and afraid.

Mrs. Bordan, an elderly lady who lives on my floor, comes to my rescue. She comes every evening, mends and irons my clothes, and tidies up my room. More importantly, she talks to me and becomes my friend. Again I am saved from deep loneliness and despair by the kindness and understanding of one person. I wonder whether Mrs. Bordan's friendship is another signpost from the Lord urging me to continue my journey.

An unpleasant experience occurs when a dinner guest in the cafeteria complains about my sloppy eating. He protests that people with my handicap should not be allowed to eat in public. This greatly embarrasses me, and I fear that the Y will evict me.

For the two and a half years I live at the Y, I keep having these "social" problems, and my presence there is a dismal social experiment. Mr. Hausmeister repeatedly complains that I ask too many favors of guests and staff. Even though I try to be independent, the elevator and restaurant doors and outside exits are just too heavy for me to manage.

Finally, when I return from my second Christmas vacation at home, there is a note in my mailbox giving me two weeks' notice to leave and stating that this is the third time I have been told to move. This is certainly news to me. I am not aware of any previous eviction notice.

I at once ask my minister, Jack Taylor, to be my advocate. He readily consents and promptly wheels me to the director's office. Jack introduces himself by saying, "I am Ruth's pastor and I am here to arbitrate your difficulties with each other. I will take no side but I want to see justice done."

When it is my turn to speak, I demand, "Why do you send me a note saying that I have been asked to move three times and have refused? The note in my hand is the first official indication that I am unwelcome." Mr. Hausmeister hems and haws and finally admits that this note is the first he has sent me.

Jack now asks the director why it is so urgent that I leave. The administrator avoids looking at me and answers Jack, "We have had so many complaints about Ruth bothering the guests by asking them for favors—opening doors and holding the elevator for her. She often interrupts our houseman when he is at work. We just cannot have this annoyance any longer. It's bad for our business."

Turning to me, Mr. Hausmeister says, "Ruth, I have an idea for you. There is a good nursing home nearby which will give you room and board while you work at HCC. They will even pack your lunch every day. Are you willing to look at it? I will take you there tomorrow morning."

I look at Jack. He nods and says quietly, "I will go with you."

So the next morning, Mr. Hausmeister drives Jack and me to a big, white clapboard house on a deserted street. When I enter my nose rebels at the urine-soaked atmosphere, and my ears hear alarming moans and groans.

A nattily dressed man introduces himself as Mr. Grundy, the home's director, and leads us through a crowded dayroom. Half-dressed people lie on the floor, and some lie on canvas hammocks, staring at the dirty ceiling. There is no meaningful activity and many patients look half-dead.

"These patients are waiting for their music appreciation hour, which will start when our activities person finishes her morning duties," Mr. Grundy explains a bit too glibly.

The director leads us to a small room which is separated from the main room only by a curtain. "This will be your room. You may do your counseling in here. Because you will do some work for us, I will reduce your bill and charge you four hundred a month instead of five hundred. Will you accept my offer?"

I look at the tiny room with a single bed, dresser, a small table, and single straight chair. I listen a moment to the cries and whimpers in the next room. I turn to Jack for an answer. He gazes at me and slowly shrugs his shoulders. I look again at the insufferable Mr. Grundy. I think, The Y wants me to get out, but I cannot come here. Conditions are so deplorable that it would be suicide.

To Mr. Grundy I say, "I will have to think about your proposal. I will call you in the morning."

As Jack and I make our way through the dreary room, a young woman patient comes up to me and says, "Don't come here. This place is a hellhole!"

All this time Mr. Hausmeister has waited in the car for us. When we get seated, he asks, "Well, how did it go? When are you going to move?"

"I'm not going to move there!" I declare. "That home is a filthy dungeon."

"Well, you better move somewhere soon!" asserts Mr. Hausmeister.

When we arrive back at the Y, Jack invites me to go to his study next door to discuss my situation. "Ruth," he begins, "you are in a tough fix. The Y will keep at you until you do move. I have an idea that may solve your problem. I know the owner of an apartment building two blocks away. I'm going to ask him if he has an efficiency or a one-bedroom apartment that you can rent. How does this strike you?"

"I will have to get someone to live with me," I reply.

Ken Follette, a counselor at HCC, hears of my plight and promptly finds someone to live with me. Deedee, an aide at HCC is a nineteen-year-old girl who is looking for a room and agrees to move in with me.

Deedee proves to be quite a responsibility. She has been raised in poverty, has little self-esteem, and lacks commonly accepted morals. We have several sharp arguments over the difference between right and wrong. We live together for eight months, during which time she helps me in return for her rent. She eventually marries her childhood sweetheart, and after the wedding, she writes me a thank-you letter for giving her a better life. Evidently, my struggles with Deedee paid off.

It is June 1969 when my mother comes to White Horse to help me look for another companion. In answer to our ad calling for a helper for a "professional person," we hire Mrs. Seddon, a widow who is nearly blind. As eccentric as she is arthritic, she nevertheless stays with me my last year at HCC.

That fall two factors indicate it is time to move. Although my salary has been raised twice, it costs more money to live in White Horse than I make. Most important, Mother wants me home. She is lonely in the big house that Dad loved.

These reasons motivate me to look for another job. I answer several ads in the *American Psychological Employment Bulletin*. Soon a letter comes from a state institution for the retarded in Pennsylvania. It is located within driving distance of Mother's home, and she is quite excited when I phone to give her the news.

When I announce my leaving at HCC, my colleagues seem genuinely sorry. My clients beg me not to go. The one I'll always remember is Robert Bourne, an African American boy. After three months at HCC, he is placed as a motel janitor. A conscientious worker, he soon is promoted to chief night janitor. In spite of a bad limp, Robert proves what a disabled person can do when motivated. He comes to see me on my last day at HCC and thanks me again and again for giving him the chance to work. Robert is my greatest success story at HCC.

On the night before my last day at work, there is a big party at HCC. After dinner, Mr. Blumegardner gives a speech thanking me for my diligent work with my clients and reminding me that I have placed thirty-five people in jobs during my three years with the agency.

Bob congratulates me on sticking to my job in spite of many problems in my living arrangements. He concludes by saying to me very directly, "Ruth, you are a good counselor. Wherever you go, whatever you do, always remember your troubles and triumphs at HCC. Those lessons will help you conquer future problems."

Bob's words prove to be true. I never forget the lessons learned at HCC. There I demonstrate to myself and others that I can hold a full-time job and that I can counsel troubled people successfully. I also experienced the warm love of my Jewish colleagues, folks whom I had known before only from a distance.

The Y also taught me a few things. Not all people tolerate the ways of the disabled. I have grown up with the expectation that those around me would grant me common courtesies, such as opening any doors. I am amazed and shocked to find that I am not always considered part of the community. I have also learned that people can be cruel.

"So you call yourself a psychologist! Humph!"

The voice from the stocky lady is harsh and sarcastic. Dr. Grace Cock, director of the Psychology Department at the State School and Hospital in Bratsworth, Pennsylvania, is interviewing me for a job. Her red, puffy face and piercing blue eyes remind me of a baboon which is ready to jump at the slightest provocation. I feel very uneasy as she proceeds to inquire about my training and recent employment. "Why did you leave your job in Wisconsin?" she asks sharply.

"I wasn't making enough money to live on," I answer, looking straight at her. "Besides, I want to live near my mother."

"What did you do at the Jew Workshop?"

"I counseled handicapped clients and prepared them for job placement."

"Did you really? I can hardly believe that. What do you think you could do here if you are employed in my department?" Dr. Cock queries disbelievingly.

I'm beginning to be irritated. I look at Mother as she shoots a warning glance at me.

"I can give performance tests, do play therapy, write reports, counsel staff, and so forth. But I'm not sure I want to," I stammer.

Here Mother cuts in. "Ruth really has done all these things. I'm sure she will be very helpful to you."

"Oh, I'm a liberal thinker. I'll give her a chance. It's not often I have a handicapped Ph.D. on my staff."

"I will have to get a housekeeper to live with me. Is there anyone in town I can hire?" I ask.

"I have a housekeeper all picked out for you," says Dr. Cock. "Belinda Schneider is one of our most responsible residents. I will send her to you in the morning." I feel it is useless to argue with the woman, so I agree to try Belinda. Mother and I make our way to the ground-floor apartment and find a pleasant six-room dwelling.

The next morning at nine, in walks a big-boned woman with hunched shoulders and a farmer's walk. "I'm Belinda and I'm wearing my new brown jumper," she announces shyly. "I'm here to help Dr. Webb and do whatever she says."

Right away Mother asks Belinda, "Can you cook?"

"Oh yes, good meals I can cook for Dr. Webb," Belinda proclaims smiling.

"Where do you come from? Are you Pennsylvania Dutch?" I ask.

"Yes, I was born in Oxford. My daddy and mother were Dutch and on their farm were living. Daddy was a truck driver with a bad heart. I was only eleven years old when he died on the operating table. Then I worked in the tobacco fields for the man who raised me when I was not in school. I can read but I can't count money."

"Well," I say, "you will have to learn to handle money because I am going to pay you twenty-five dollars a week and I want you to save ten dollars every week to put in your savings account."

Under Mother's guidance, Belinda learns to prepare my dinner and clean the apartment. After a month, Belinda learns to use the telephone to make a beauty shop appointment for herself. I lavish great praise on her, and she practically glows with happiness.

Meanwhile, in getting acquainted with Dr. Cock, it takes only a couple of days before I realize that she tightly controls the activities of her two master's-degree assistants, who periodically test the more than four hundred profoundly retarded patients.

My expectations that I will have a vital and challenging job are quickly dashed. Apparently Dr. Cock does not think I can do anything on my own and does not assign me any patients to test or any reports to write. My suggestion that I visit patients and write reports is ignored. She forbids me to attend weekly staff meetings, saying that the ancient elevator is too unreliable for me to operate. In fact, Dr. Cock seems afraid to let me go to the wards and talk with other staff. This isolation from other hospital professionals humiliates and infuriates me from the very beginning of my employment at Bratsworth. I do not protest for fear of losing control of my growing anger.

One day Dr. Cock is absent and I am asked to test a new admission. I am overwhelmed with fear that I will do something displeasing to my boss. I give the ten-year-old boy the Grace Arthur Performance Scale, a test which I had used at HCC. When the choleric Dr. Cock sees my report the next day, she explodes in scornful criticism. After her reprimand, I feel like sinking into the floor.

One morning, Superintendent Fetters comes into my office and announces that he is appointing me director of research. I look at Dr. Cock's face and see that she is not at all pleased. After Dr. Fetters leaves, she loses no time in telling me that I will never see a research project. As a matter of fact, she is working on a grant application for a new Education Department. I never get to see her plans.

To provide respite from my gloom in the Psychology Department, several speech and occupational therapists invite Belinda and me on all-day excursions to the town of Hershey and to Gettysburg. These trips provide escape from the tension and stress of Dr. Cock's office. When Dr. Cock hears about our excursions, she frowns and exclaims, "Dr. Webb, you shouldn't waste your time with people who are not psychologists!"

Agnes Murphy, the institution's physical therapist, and I hit it off right away. She is interested in my sensory motor training and invites me to collaborate with her in a pilot study with five profoundly retarded children. Using the knowledge I gained from Dr. McCallister in White Horse, I formulate a program of exercises to evoke motor responses in these severely handicapped children to sights, sounds, smells, and tastes.

In spite of Dr. Cock's disparaging remarks that the profoundly retarded can never improve, Agnes and I plan a six-month program in which we devote an hour a day to five children.

Before the end of the six-months-long project, the children, who have been unable to grasp toys or food, begin to hold cookies and take them to their mouths. The ward staff members are elated over their progress and compliment our efforts. Everyone but Dr. Cock is pleased. Little do I then realize that this pilot study is to give me background experience in my later work with perceptual motor training of retarded children.

About three months after my arrival at Bratsworth, I begin to have terrible headaches. Every Saturday morning I wake up with a blinding, throbbing pain across my forehead. It takes the entire day for the pain to ease. The next day I am tired and worn out.

Every other weekend an obliging maintenance man from the hospital drives Belinda and me to visit Mother. One Sunday when I am at home, Mother and I visit an old friend, who takes one look at my drooping mouth and asks, "What is the matter with you, Ruth?"

Mother quickly answers, "Ruth is having a hard time with her boss at work. She is so unfair and critical to Ruth. I don't know what to do."

Our friend replies in a loud whisper, "Get Ruth out of that place. Quick! Before she has a nervous breakdown."

Mother nods, "I'll do what I can, as soon as I can!"

One Friday evening there is a knock at the door. When Belinda opens it, my old friend Robert Clayton enters and announces that he is on a weekend sales trip to the Pennsylvania Dutch country for Allstate Insurance Company. May he stay overnight with us?

I invite him in, and Belinda shows him the guest room. After he takes his bags to the room, he comes out into the living room and we talk for three hours. He tells me that his wife, Mildred, nags him unmercifully because he does not have a secure job.

My guest talks so long that Belinda goes to bed and falls asleep. At 10:30, I yawn and say, "Robert, I think I'm going to bed. What about you?" Robert says okay and goes to his room.

I go into the bathroom and take off my blouse. Robert enters and, without a word, puts on my nightgown and then carries me into my bed. Undressing himself to the skin, he asks me, "Have you ever had sexual relations before?"

Dazed, I shake my head, "No."

"Well, I'm going to show you how it feels. You can't be a real woman without having sex."

He then proceeds to penetrate me very gently and very lovingly. When his act is over, he says, "Now you know what sex is. I didn't want you to go through life without knowing."

By this time, I am bewildered, but I do not have any resentment of Robert. I sense he means me no harm. My feelings are so submerged that I feel no fear. I do not mention the escapade to anyone for a long, long time. I often ponder the meaning of this experience and cannot read its meaning for my journey. I finally realize that Robert had indeed broadened my experience and had made me more of a "real woman"! But for three months thereafter, I look fearfully for signs of my being pregnant.

All this time, I have a daily battle with Dr. Cock. When the day begins, she summons me to her office to review her tasks for the day. My invited comments invariably evoke her angry reply. She gives me the impression that my opinion is not worth much, but yet she continues to request my advice. One morning I have the courage to ask, "Dr. Cock, when you hired me, what did you expect me to do? I'm tired of doing nothing!"

Her face turns red and she does not answer for a moment. Then she remarks, "Dr. Webb, your recommendation from Wisconsin claims that you can counsel clients, give tests, and write worthy reports. I have not seen you do these things. I don't think you are capable of discharging the duties of a psychologist. I know Dr. Fetters thinks you can do research, but I have grave doubts that you can even write a simple psychological report."

"Dr. Cock," I interrupt heatedly, "you haven't given me a chance to show you what I can do. Mostly I sit in my office and read all day and talk to you. But I am doing psychological research with Agnes Murphy."

"What you two are doing is *not* psychological research. You will never get improvement in those profoundly retarded children!"

Soon after this conversation, I take our friend's advice to heart to seek a new job. I don't think I can stay much longer with Dr. Cock, so I decide to tell her I'm looking for another job and ask for her secretary's help to write application letters for me.

Dr. Cock surprises me by quickly agreeing to let Judy, the department secretary, write letters for me. For three months, I pore over the monthly *Employment Bulletin* of the American Psychological Association. Every month, I select twelve or more agencies which are advertising for psychologists, and Judy obligingly sends a letter to them.

One day when Mother is visiting me, Dr. Cock invites her to her office for a so-called chat. My boss abruptly warns my mother, "Ruth is courting disaster by seeking a job she cannot do. Don't let her have a tragic failure."

When Mother tells me about Dr. Cock's opinion, I explode with anger. I wheel immediately into the director's office and declare, "Dr. Cock, you are not to discuss my plans with my mother. I deeply resent your interference in my affairs. I am old enough to make my own decisions!"

Without blinking an eye, Dr. Cock murmurs innocently, "Your mother and I were just having a friendly chat."

Early in August 1967, I get a letter from a Dr. William Peabody in Red Wing, Iowa, offering me a job as a team psychologist at the state institution for the retarded. The job pays $12,500, which is $1,000 more than I am making.

When I call Mother and tell her about the offer, she is less than pleased. "I don't want you to be so far away," she tells me.

I am in a quandary. This job seems to be a great opportunity. It offers more money and freedom to do worthwhile work. But Mother is alone and needs me. It is a terrible wrench for both of us to live so far away from each other. What should I do?

That night I write Dr. Peabody that I am very sorry but I cannot accept his offer. Two days later an airmail letter arrives from Iowa and informs me that if I accept the job, my salary will be raised by $1,000.

I still hesitate. Can Mother get along without me? Can I take Belinda? I need advice. I call my old friend, the Rev. Joe Bishop.

The next day Joe arrives at my door and says, "I have come to see for myself what is going on here with you and your boss."

After meeting Dr. Cock and listening to her voice from my office, Joe agrees that I am having a hard time at Bratsworth and concludes, "Ruth, you better find another job before that woman makes you sick. There must be other institutions where people would appreciate your gifts. Don't waste yourself by staying here."

When I tell Joe that I have turned down the job at Red Wing, he says very emphatically, "Ruth, you get on the phone and tell that man that you accept his offer. You want to escape Dr. Cock's clutches, don't you?" This question spurs me to call the Red Wing Institute. Only Joe could have changed my mind.

I call Dr. Peabody the next morning and tell him that I accept the job. He is delighted and wants me to come at once. However, before finalizing our agreement, I tell him that I would like to visit the Red Wing institution. Dr. Peabody assents, and we arrange a visit for the next Monday morning.

Belinda hears that I am thinking of moving and becomes very upset because she does not want me to leave her. I assure her that if I go, I will take her with me, but she is not convinced. She is very afraid that she will be abandoned again.

I fly out to Des Moines, Iowa, on TWA Sunday evening and am

met by Anna Seasons from the Red Wing Institute. She drives me to the institute and introduces me to Dr. Peabody, who interrupts his Sunday to meet me.

Dr. Peabody questions me about my experience with the mentally retarded and remarks that I am applying for a job in Iowa at the right time because the state has just launched a "hire the handicapped" campaign (I always wonder if one of my spirit guides arranged this timing).

During supper in the institute's cafeteria, Anna tells me that the main job of the eight psychologists is to do routine testing of the Red Wing population and to act as team psychologists for the various living areas.

I spend the next morning on the ward where the profoundly retarded live. I watch staff try to stimulate eye-hand coordination by shaking colored rattles and bells in front of the children as they lie in beanbag chairs. I am impressed by their attitude that even the most severely handicapped child can learn.

When I return to Dr. Peabody's office, he asks, "Well, Dr. Webb, will you consider a position as one of our psychologists? With your background, I think you will be able to help us in our research project to develop training techniques for the profoundly retarded. Are you interested?"

"Yes, I am," I say excitedly. "But first I have a question. May I bring the Bratsworth resident who is helping me to Red Wing?"

"I will have to ask Dr. Leach, our superintendent, about that. Both Iowa and Pennsylvania will have to approve. I will let you know before you leave this afternoon."

My plane to Philadelphia leaves at two o'clock, so there is just time for me to eat lunch and drive to the airport. On the way, Anna tells me that Belinda's transfer to Iowa has been approved.

There is no doubt that Belinda is glad to see me. I tell her that I have another job in Iowa and she cries, "Are you going to leave me?"

"Belinda, I'm going to ask Dr. Clayton to let you go with me. Don't be afraid. Everything will turn out all right."

That weekend Belinda and I go home to visit Mother, who is eager to hear about my trip to Red Wing. While we are there, another spirit-led coincidence occurs. Sunday after church I meet Benny Johnson, a friend from my YAGs days. "Why are you looking so glum?" he asks. I tell him about my hostile boss and he exclaims, "Ruth, I think something must be done about this. You are too valuable a person to be wasted. I am going to write your superintendent. What is his name?" I try to stop him from doing this, but he will not listen. So with great trepidation, I await Dr. Cock's explosion.

I want Dr. Fetters to know my plans before Dr. Cock hears them. To be sure that my conversation is private, I phone the superintendent at his home on Sunday evening. He immediately comes over to my kitchen and I tell him about the offer from Red Wing and that I want to take Belinda with me.

Dr. Fetters is silent for a moment. Then he says, "Ruth, I hate to lose you, but I know that Dr. Cock will not permit you to advance here. You'd better take this opportunity while it's here. I'm sure there will be a transfer for Belinda. After a year, if she makes good as your housekeeper, we will discharge her permanently."

"Thank you, Dr. Fetters!" I exclaim, while catching a glimpse of Belinda standing behind the door into the living room. "I will treat her as my own daughter."

"I will call a meeting tomorrow and invite you and Belinda, Dr. Cock, the head nurse, and our social worker to discuss a conditional discharge for this lady," Dr. Fetters concludes.

The next morning Dr. Cock is ill and does not come to work for two days. Judy tells me that she has a bad case of colitis. I learn then that Dr. Cock's friends in Superintendent Fetters's office have passed Benny's letter to her. And Dr. Cock's gastrointestinal tract has indeed reacted violently to Benny's protest.

Dr. Fetters waits no longer, and on the third morning, he calls the meeting in his office without Dr. Cock. Everyone but Mr. Tulip, the social worker, enthusiastically supports my request to take Belinda to Iowa.

When asked, Belinda makes it very clear that she wants to come with me. She utterly rejects a proposal to place her as an attendant in a nursing home. Belinda emphatically declares, "I've had enough of taking care of babies!"

Belinda and I are then asked to leave the room while the committee makes a decision. We wait for only five minutes until Dr. Clayton calls us back into the conference room and announces, "Dr. Webb, Belinda is free to go with you. We are very impressed with the care you have given her."

When Dr. Cock returns the next day, she says to me, "I understand that funny things are going on here in my absence. When are you leaving?"

"I plan to leave the second of September and to spend two weeks with my Mother. I start my new job at Red Wing on September 15th, 1967."

"Then you will leave this Friday. I certainly hope you will find work you can do and that you are not overestimating your ability to work in an institution. You have not shown this capability here."

I open my mouth to answer but no words come.

"We will have to have a going-away party for you. How about next Thursday afternoon? I will invite all the department heads."

"Will you give me a written evaluation before I leave?" I ask this question because I have become very suspicious of Dr. Cock. I do not want to leave and give her the opportunity to place an unfavorable performance rating in my record without giving me the chance to refute it.

This is Monday. I wait until Wednesday morning before reminding Dr. Cock again of my evaluation. When she hesitates, I go to Mr. Cornwallis, the personnel director, and demand that I receive an evaluation. Finally on Thursday morning, he presents me with a mildly critical evaluation from Dr. Cock. Her main complaint is that I do not keep busy and that I do not look for work to do.

In my reply to Dr. Cock's criticism, I state that I have not been assigned any duties in my field of expertise, i.e., writing research grants and counseling.

An hour before the party, I take off for my last round of the hospital wards to say good-by to the nurses whom I have come to know and respect. I visit the ward with the four-year-old Siamese twins who are joined at the chest and say hello to small children with twisted limbs and staring eyes.

Dr. Cock's voice suddenly blares out from the loudspeaker, "Dr. Webb, Dr. Webb, come to your office immediately!"

I do not move at once but say good-by to my favorite patients, the members of our sensory motor project. They have aroused a hope in me that I can help severely retarded people learn by teaching them to move in response to sensory stimulation.

When I do arrive at the psychology office, I find my mother, Belinda, and almost all the professional staff of the institution. My friend Agnes Murphy hurries in and whispers, "I did not want to come before you were here because I can't stand your director."

"Dr. Webb, we are waiting for you," Dr. Cock asserts. "All our professionals are here. Now I can bring the cake in." She disappears into the kitchen and brings out a white cake with a three foot diameter, decorated with pink and green flowers. Placing it in front of me, she says, "Dr. Webb, I had this cake baked especially for you. I hope you will always remember your colleagues at Bratsworth."

Mother's eyes are as big as saucers. When we are at last alone, she asks me, "Ruth, do you think the size of that cake has any relation to Dr. Cock's guilty conscience?"

The next morning Belinda and I leave Bratsworth State School and Hospital forever. As we drive out of the gate, I try to evaluate my experience there. I reason, Dr. Cock showed me how an angry person can manipulate others to inflate her own ego. She hired me for the sole purpose of congratulating herself for helping a poor cripple. When I proved to be more capable than she imagined, she became afraid that I would overshadow her and began to belittle me at every opportunity.

My job at Bratsworth has given me a different kind of rejection than I experienced in White Horse. There I was successful in performing my professional duties but persecuted in my living environment. At Bratsworth, professional status and satisfaction in discharging acknowledged duties were denied to me, whereas my home life was relatively undisturbed. Dr. Cock did bequeath one valuable gift to me. My life is indeed enhanced by the challenge of caring for Belinda.

9

Mountains and Valleys
in Red Wing

"Welcome to Red Wing!"

The gray-haired lady holds open the heavy door. "You are the new psychologist and her friend, Belinda. I am Emma Hammerstone, social worker in Area 5. I think you are assigned to our area. Let me take your bags."

She grabs a heavy suitcase in each hand with the comment, "I'm used to toting bags for my son on his home visits. He lives here in the cottage for young men with Down's syndrome."

"I am surprised that Red Wing patients can go home," I murmur.

"Oh yes, I take Russell home every weekend I'm not on duty. You take the elevator there on the right, and I'll meet you on the second floor, where our guest apartment is located."

So saying, Mrs. Hammerstone quickly disappears upstairs. When the elevator opens, the friendly social worker leads us down a long hall to a suite of rooms, which includes a bedroom, bath, and sitting room, all gaily decorated with orange and brown rugs.

When we are alone, Belinda again exclaims, "Dr. Webb, this is a nice room but when will we have our own home? I don't want to live here! It's too much like my old institution." Throughout the two weeks we live in this apartment, Belinda keeps worrying that we will not get our own home.

I contact a realtor, and on our second Friday, she locates a little red ranch home on a quiet street in Red Wing, which I can rent for $250 a month. When we go to look at it that evening, we find it is ideally suited to our needs.

There is a big living room with a picture window at the front of the house. A dinette and kitchen overlook the backyard, which is a large enough hunting ground for two dogs. The house has three bedrooms, one of which is master-bedroom size. A basement and attic are included.

The little red house is just what I need. It requires a few alterations—a ramp at the back door, a strong rail over the bath tub, and later when I own it, a window near the dining table, bookcases in my den, a fire escape door in my bedroom, and a room for Mother.

A year passes, and our landlord offers to sell me the house for $14,500. While I am considering his offer, there is a knock on the door one Saturday morning. Mother, who happens to be visiting, opens the door to see a smiling gentleman.

"Hello, I am Bert Aldrich, Red Wing's best realtor. I understand that you would like to buy this house. I would like to help you procure the deed to the property, etc."

Mother always says that the Lord sent Mr. Aldrich to my door that day. Whether it is the Lord's doing or just Mr. Aldrich's shrewdness in sniffing out a deal, I don't know. I am thrilled to have my own home. To show my affection for it, I keep it painted red, my favorite color. For me, owning the "Little Red House" is an irrefutable mark of personhood.

Our house is five blocks from the typical Iowa town square, which is easy walking distance for Belinda to push me in my light-weight wheelchair. A pharmacy, two hardware stores, a furniture store, beauty shop, and grocery surround the large, grassy plot on which the county courthouse stands.

One block before we reach the town square is "church row," where four churches are situated. I am destined to belong to two of these churches. In the first, I meet rejection from the pastor, who cannot seem to reconcile my possession of both a Ph.D. and cerebral palsy. He struggles with my name every time he greets me. One Sunday he calls me Ruth and the next week I am Dr. Webb. Because he is so obviously uncomfortable in my presence and cannot accept me as a person, I finally leave the church.

The second church has a small congregation which completely accepts me. Its minister, the Rev. Carl, visits me each week and brings me Bible lessons. He invites me to join the church council. Belinda and I attend many church potlucks, annual meetings, and state conferences. We both feel welcomed by the congregation.

Red Wing is a friendly town, and Belinda soon learns to greet the various merchants by name as she enters their places of business. They reciprocate by calling her Lindy, and this recognition makes her face glow with happiness. Belinda really feels accepted in Red Wing and considers it her own hometown.

I am delighted to see Belinda blossoming in all kinds of ways. When we first met at Bratsworth, Belinda was afraid to make a phone call, make change, shop, or plan a meal. Some five years later, although hesitant in new situations, she is quite competent in routine duties, such as using a washing machine, vacuuming, and making beds.

When well, Belinda is loving, kind, and talkative. She is very loyal and concerned about me. She enjoys celebrations, especially Christmas, and is delighted when she can help trim the tree.

Belinda enjoys grocery shopping and learning to cook. This love for food is nearly her undoing. Her doctor warns her that her weight is contributing to her very high blood pressure and migraines and may lead to a stroke. However, Belinda continues to eat as if she is still a farmhand. We try many diets to decrease her weight and migraines. They all are initially successful, but after a few weeks, Belinda grows tired of them, begins to gain weight again, and then refuses to cooperate any longer.

With her painful migraines come periods of severe depression. When Belinda is hurting, she is very irritable and prone to temper tantrums. Her crying may last from one to five minutes. At these times, she is easily frustrated, and her anger is projected on me as torrents of "nasty words" tumble from her tongue. After a moment, Belinda recovers and asks for my forgiveness. During these episodes, my feelings are sometimes so badly hurt that I lash out at Belinda. Then we both cry because I too burst into tears when I get angry.

Soon after our arrival in Red Wing, kindly old Dr. Steel declares that since Belinda has had no seizures for five years, she has no further need of Dilantin (an antiseizure drug). Seven years pass before she again has seizures, which start in her left arm, travel down to her legs, and up again into her right arm.

Eventually, an ingenious physician explains her many problems. He says that Belinda's unconscious mind converts her underlying anxiety into physical symptoms such as colds, seizures, and migraines. From then on, Belinda discards her symptoms one by one and becomes more self-assured. One day Belinda sums up her happiness by saying, "Dr. Webb, I love you. I don't ever want to leave. I don't ever want to leave you or the little red house!"

My work at the Red Wing Institute progresses well for the first four years. It is my good fortune to arrive at Red Wing on September 16, 1967. At the peak of national interest in the mentally retarded, I have a job as team psychologist for that multiple-handicapped group.

I am given responsibility for ten wards, and I try hard to get acquainted with the patients in them. As I slowly guide my motor chair between the rows of white cribs, I try to evoke a smile or wave of a limp hand from the little ones behind the crib bars.

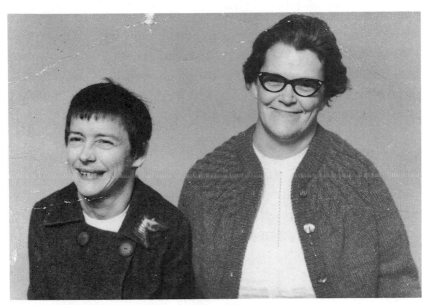

Ruth Cameron Webb and Belinda Schneider, Red Wing, Iowa, 1972

Some lie still, unable to move their rigid limbs. Others display hyperactivity, which causes them to constantly move their arms, legs, and heads every moment they are awake. Those who are ambulatory require close supervision so that they do not leave the ward unattended.

As I roam these wards of human outcasts, I find a small number of individuals who are terribly physically handicapped but yet respond to words and smiles from the staff. By gesturing, some express their likes and dislikes in regard to food, clothes, and television programs. I later discover that such individuals make up about 1 percent of the institutionalized retarded in the United States. I fervently resolve to help these persons at Red Wing.

Red Wing has a Hospital Improvement Program (HIP) grant for the pediatric ward in Blackwood Hall. Its mandate is to develop improved methods of care for profoundly retarded people. In conjunction with this grant, the nursing staff and administration are looking for a program to improve the learning capacity of their profoundly retarded children. With the sensory motor techniques from White Horse, I am at the right place at the right time.

When Lucy Black, R.N., the director of the HIP program, hears about my interest in sensory motor training, she eagerly incorporates my sensory motor exercises into her HIP program and has me teach training techniques to her staff.

Drawing on my knowledge gained from Dr. McCallister in Wisconsin and from my experience with the pilot study at Bratsworth, I design a program to test the effectiveness of sensory stimulation and passive gross and fine motor exercises on ten HIP grant youngsters. I coin the term *Developmental Therapy* to include sensory motor techniques used to promote awareness (reaction to sights, sounds, touch, smells, and tastes), manipulation (manual dexterity and social interaction), and posture (sitting, standing, and walking).

With assistance from Janet Strong, a special education teacher, I select experimental and control groups, each with five children. Each group includes three girls and two boys, ages four to ten. A brother is assigned to the E group and his sister is a member of the C group. All have severe motor handicaps caused by trauma or injury and I.Q.'s below ten.

After six months, our results indicate that the experimental group has gained in awareness and manipulation while the control group shows no change. All in the E group respond to their names and look at noisemakers. Two children reach for and hold small toys. Each responds by looking toward the record player when the nursery rhymes are played to begin the daily training session. These improvements are not seen in the control group.

I receive many compliments on the 2 East sensory motor program from Dan Smith, my first program administrator. He is a social worker and a very decent gentleman. He encourages me to enlarge my program. Dan and I have many talks about my hope that sensory motor stimulation will improve learning ability in profoundly retarded youngsters.

Every morning Janet and I work with individual children, putting them through passive arm and leg movements and encouraging "visual pursuit," hand reaching, and grasping by waving noisemakers and gaily colored windmills from left to right in front of them.

Three-year-old Charlie is our first Red Wing success. He is as limp as a rag doll when we begin to work with him. He cannot sit up by himself and can barely hold toys. After six months of sensory motor training, Charlie can sit up, hold and transfer toys from one hand to the other, and is beginning to pull himself up in his crib. As time passes, he learns to walk and advances to the so-called trainable range of mental retardation.

Besides my work with Lucy Black and the HIP Program, I am kept busy recording progress and writing annual reports on all 180 residents of Blackwood Hall. I try to visit each of the ten wards every day. I am busy and happy at this stage of my journey. I am finally doing a worthwhile job.

1970 is a very eventful year. Mr. Melon, superintendent, makes me director of developmental therapy. I and my therapists design The Awareness, Manipulation and Posture Index I (and later AMP II and AMP III for severely and moderately retarded children) as a pre-post training evaluation instrument for young children in the entire range of retardation. I publish five articles on sensory motor training of the profoundly retarded as measured by the AMP I—the first four on training profoundly retarded children and the fifth on working with adults.

For four years, the Developmental Therapy Department flourishes. There are fourteen therapists, including Janet Strong, the program coordinator. We work in all five areas of the institution, and at one time, we have a case load of 204 patients.

Our department records show that a third of our trainees under ten years improve markedly after two years of sensory motor training. Another third improve slightly, while the remaining third do not improve at all. This ratio is identical to the success rate reported in the literature for other therapies.

The AMP Index brings many visitors to observe our techniques. Requests for information on sensory motor training come from countries such as England, Holland, Germany, and India, as well as from many places in the United States.

The AMP makes me so well known in Iowa that the Governor's Committee on Employment of the Handicapped selects me as the Handicapped Iowan of 1971. In March, I am the guest of honor at the governor's dinner in a Des Moines hotel. There is a steak dinner, wine, music, and a speech by the governor lauding me for my work with the profoundly retarded and awarding me a huge gold plaque.

I respond by speaking as clearly as I can, saying, "Thank you for this great honor. Credit for these achievements is not wholly mine but belongs to my parents, to the many who have helped me along the way, and to my Lord."

At this time, I do not know that this is the most climactic moment in my career. This night my dreams of making a significant contribution seem to come true. I am overjoyed.

This is supposed to be my time to shine. But my seventy-nine-year-old mother, who has come west for this special occasion, steals the spotlight. Very elated that her daughter is being honored, she wears a dark, kelly green, satin dress and flits around like a teenager. In my fifty years of knowing Mother, I cannot remember a time when she is as excited as she is now.

All this time, my acquaintance with Anna Seasons, who made me so welcome on my first trip to Red Wing and who now is a county official, grows into a firm friendship. She spends many Saturday evenings with Belinda and me playing Scrabble and in addition, takes us monthly to a play or symphony concert. Eating out is a real treat for Belinda and me, and we relish the many fine eateries.

Unfortunately, the previous September my mother came down with a severe case of shingles at her home in Pennsylvania. One morning she woke with great pain from large blisters on her left shoulder, under her arm, and on her left breast. Mother is to live

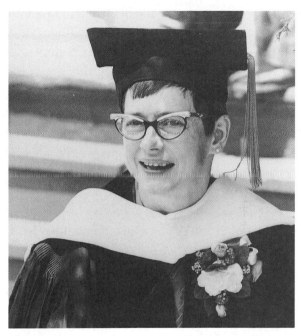

*Ruth Cameron Webb, receiving Doctor of Humane
Letters honorary degree from Drew University, 1978*

nine and a half years with the searing, itching, and aching pain of
shingles. Five of these years she lives alone in the big, family house,
and although she endures ever-increasing pain, she continues to
drive her car.

At last, in October 1977, Mother consents to my wish that she sell
the house and move permanently to Red Wing. I am relieved that
she is no longer alone and proud that I can take care of her. I consider this to be a privilege and responsibility of personhood.

To my great consternation, Belinda and Mother never get along.
Mother cannot tolerate Belinda's slowness. Belinda cannot take her
constant criticism and disapproval. Each brings the other to tears
at times. This sparring is worse when I am at work and can do
nothing to help the situation.

An unexpected honor for me comes in May 1978, when my alma
mater, Drew University, awards me the honorary degree of Doctor

of Humane Letters. Mother, in a wheelchair, David and Frances, Aunts Ethel and Louise, the Rev. Joe, and Belinda are all there to hear my beloved professor, Dr. Mac, read my commendation.

The day after my return from receiving this honor for my work, I learn that the Red Wing Institute has abolished all departments. Area administrators are now in charge of all professional services. My developmental therapists are assigned to one of the five residential areas and take orders from a nonspecialist administrator.

I am highly indignant over the way my four years of pioneer work are ruthlessly destroyed by someone's unknowing and apparently uncaring pen. And no one is considerate enough to give me the reasons for the elimination of the Developmental Therapy Department. I seethe with anger for a long time.

Regardless of my feelings, the change comes. My authority is drained away. One administrator forbids me to enter his area to supervise my therapist. Another forbids the therapists in his area to attend our Friday-afternoon departmental meetings, which I consider essential in educating therapists who are high school graduates.

I face a highly emotional crisis in Area 5. Red-haired Damon Rust, the Area 5 administrator, comes thundering into the developmental wards.

He then shouts at me, "Dr. Webb, your developmental therapy is a bunch of words, a hoax! I don't want you on my staff. I'm letting you on my team only because Mr. Melon has ordered me to do so."

Damon's hatred for me is undisguised. He does not assign me any duties. I sit in my office all day long and remember my experience with Dr. Cock at Bratsworth. Although I fear greatly for my job, I determine not to give him cause to fire me. I spend seven miserable days as an Area 5 psychologist without portfolio.

Then a miracle happens. Within two weeks of his promotion, Damon leaves his administrative post at Red Wing. Rumors fly that he is fired for misconduct. At any rate, I am relieved from another experience of working with one who does not like me.

Then begins my ordeal with Martha Smothers. She is an old Army nurse, accustomed to command. My cerebral palsy bothers her. She acts as if I should be a patient instead of a psychologist. In the three years I work with her, she never relates to me as a colleague.

My first unpleasant encounter with this unpredictable lady comes when she trips angrily and rapidly down the hall to my office and accuses me of saying she is senile. Several weeks later, Martha declares that I open mail belonging to Donna Morgan, the other psychologist in Area 5. Her accusation stems from my innocent act of picking up from Donna's desk an announcement of a university seminar on depression.

The next day I receive a memo in which Martha accuses me of reading Donna's mail, listening to Donna's phone conversations (our phones are on the same line), and asking too many favors of Donna. I am too shaken to wonder how Martha knows what transpires in our psychology office. Martha also accuses me of not doing my job. I wonder if she ever reads the volumes of reports I write or the progress notes and ward observations I record.

Donna advises me to reply point by point in a memo to Martha with a copy to Mr. Melon. The next day Mr. Melon writes me a return memo congratulating me on my defense and saying that my memo will be placed in my personnel file along with Martha's memo. I read my personnel record before my retirement and find Martha's memo, but my rebuttal is missing.

Martha comes to my office for a last time just before her retirement and vehemently denies that she does not like me. I know, however, that she cannot overcome the "psychosomatic effect," i.e., a stranger's reactions on seeing a disabled person.

When the Iowa Board of Education visits the institute, a board member interviews me about my job. I venture to tell him how Martha is treating me. The gentleman readily promises to investigate the situation without betraying my confidence.

He asks Mortimer Feathers, director of special education, to corroborate my complaints. Dr. Feathers substantiates my report to the board and informs Superintendent Melon of my plight.

At this juncture, on December 11, 1980, a rubber brush wears out on my motor chair. The motor misfires and the chair goes forward when I try to reverse. I happen to be near the stairs on the first floor, and so I and my chair bump down thirteen steps and tip over on the landing leading to the basement. During that wild, noisy ride, I keep wondering what will happen when I reach the bottom step.

It takes only a minute to find out. I am knocked out and suffer a concussion and a broken wrist. I spend five days in the hospital and eight weeks at home. Mother is with us at the time, and so I gain a nice visit with her as an extra bonus from my ride down the stairs.

During my convalescence, I negotiate with Dr. Feathers for a position in the institute's Department of Special Education. He knows me by my developmental therapy reputation. At a workshop he has seen my switch, operated by hand or foot and designed to enable severely disabled children to change slides whenever they wish. Repeated reflection on our conversation and ensuing events make me wonder which of my spirit guides was near at that meeting.

For when I return to work, Dr. Feathers has me transferred to the special education department. Mortimer Feathers later tells me that he believes God sent him to Red Wing to rescue me from Area 5. His remark makes me wonder if my ride down thirteen steps is part of the Lord's rescue plan or just a convenient coincidence to introduce me to another spirit guide.

Mort tells me to observe the classrooms and let the teachers get acquainted with me. He then has me collect ideas for a new curriculum. So I proceed to build a curriculum for students who are profoundly and severely retarded, trainable, and educable. I then devise a three-level academic evaluation to correspond with the curriculum. Finally, I write a perceptual motor training program for the Learning Clinic Dr. Feathers and I are planning.

The Learning Clinic is progressing well, and I am very satisfied

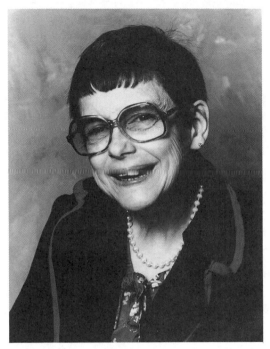

Ruth Cameron Webb, Red Wing, Iowa, c. 1980

with its results. However, three days before Christmas 1980, Mother and I are having a heated discussion over a long-forgotten issue when she turns toward me, twists her body, and falls and breaks her hip. I will always remember her look that says, "This is the end."

I visit Mother twice a week in the hospital, where they pin her hip. Her left leg has poor circulation and becomes black and she cannot walk. It is out of the question for Belinda to care for her in the little red house.

I decide to put Mother in the nursing home in Red Wing, where I can visit every afternoon after work. Mother does not like the home, and every morning she has me phone Barb, the head nurse, about this-and-that staff error, e.g., not giving her coffee for breakfast, or not sending her to physical therapy, etc. Mother deteriorates fast. Her left leg is so gangrenous that the physical therapist cannot stand her up. She then catches pneumonia and is very miserable.

A month later, my friend Opal and I arrive at the nursing home around 4:10 P.M. We chat with Barb, the head nurse, for about five minutes. She has just given Mother her medicine and reports that Mother is alert.

When we enter her room, Mother's eyes are closed and she is breathing noisily. Opal goes immediately for help as I continue to watch Mother. Opal returns and reports that Barb will come when she finishes giving medicines. Mother continues her labored breathing.

While Opal goes for the nurse a second time, Mother nods her head up and down, as is her custom when agreeing with someone, and breathes her last. I am sure that Dad is there to greet her at her passing.

The next moment the nurses come running. They shove me out of the room, bring an oxygen tank, and try to revive Mother, but to no avail. Dr. Steel comes quickly and gravely tells me, "She has expired."

My brother David hurries out for the memorial service at the church. I never cry throughout the funeral preparations, during the memorial service, or the next day when David throws away her things. My brother breaks down and weeps during the service.

My friend Anna tells me I am deeply relieved that Mother is free from pain. She asserts that I have seen Mother suffer too much to cry. But I did grieve, and I still do.

I will always remember that the many struggles to become independent from Mother were great hurdles on my journey into personhood. She loved me so much that she could not break the habit of overprotecting me.

Although I often rebelled against my close dependence on her, Mother's loving persistence and faith in my learning abilities led me to start my journey in the first place and to continue it over very rough terrain. I owe Mother much—the will to struggle and to achieve my goal of personhood. Even today, I often feel her presence, especially at night.

For four years now, I have been growing more and more depressed. Mother's shingles, Belinda's migraines, and the continuing no-win situation at work all converge on me at once and keep increasing in severity. These troubles are more than I can handle.

My young pastor finds help for me in Dorothy Bradley, a Christian counselor. After reading my early journal, Dorothy observes that I have been depressed for most of my life because of cerebral palsy. Although I have long realized this, it is tremendously comforting to have her state the issue so matter-of-factly.

Dorothy pulls me out of depression through counseling, prayer, and meditation. The lessons I learn from this wise spirit guide are invaluable. To stay healthy mentally, I must maintain a daily time of prayer and meditation. When I skip a day or two, I begin to be discouraged.

Dorothy suggests that I attend the charismatic prayer meetings at St. Margaret Mary's Catholic Church in Omaha. Martina, my doctor's wife, drives Belinda and me to the meetings. The songs and talks during those evenings give me welcome relief from my depression. These meetings probably save me from a complete breakdown.

As the memory of Mother's death recedes in time, I am grateful to be able to thrust my energies into the Learning Clinic. Dr. Feathers sends Sarah King, who is belatedly getting her teacher's certificate, to assist me. She works with me for three years and helps me prepare materials for an educational assessment on three levels. Half our time is spent doing academic evaluations and half in sensory and perceptual motor training. We work with children and adolescents whose learning difficulties cause behavior problems.

I am especially fond of a group of four young men in their late teens. Each one is notorious for losing his temper and becoming violent. They all have reading problems and motor uncoordination; none of them can step heel-to-toe on a line painted on the floor or level a two-foot-wide balance board as it stands on a one-inch keel. Some find it difficult to match words and numbers.

Once a week we have "Blow-Outs" time. We discuss out-of-control situations which have happened during the week. Gradually these young men learn to express their frustrations verbally and to plan more satisfying ways to vent their anger.

In its zenith, the Learning Clinic sees sixteen students three times a week for remediation of learning and emotional problems. I feel proud when I remember how we help some students, especially with reading. Both Sarah and I are happy to have these successes.

When Sarah receives her teaching certificate, she leaves me for a better job. I am never given a replacement for her because of budget constraints. Without an aide, I cannot continue sensory motor training and resign myself to write an annual educational assessment report on each of our 150 students. Year after year, I give the same level assessments to nearly the same students.

After three or four years of getting almost identical results, I become bored, as do the teachers who now are obliged to assist me in giving their students the assessment. When eight years pass, I am so frustrated with my testing program that right after my sixty-fourth birthday, I resign from the Red Wing Institute.

As my retirement approaches, I remember a conversation with Mr. Melon about my theory of developmental therapy. He seemed to imply that I do not offer a plausible rationale for my sensory motor exercises. At that time, I tell him that my awareness, manipulation, and posture theory is based upon observed dysfunctions exhibited by the profoundly retarded.

With this memory in mind, I become more and more determined to find out the truth as to why my Developmental Therapy Department was so surreptitiously disbanded. Was it really because I lacked a clearly defined theory? What part did my own personality play in the demise of my "great achievement" in life? Did the department fall because I, a disabled female, had gained too much fame from abroad and so had incurred the jealousy of my colleagues?

When I ask Superintendent Melon what happened to the department, he acts surprised. "Isn't the developmental therapy program being carried out in the living areas under the program administrators? Aren't you still the director of D.T. and don't you represent the department on my advisory committee?" he queries.

I answer, "The D.T. Department exists only on paper. The program administrators don't have the program and they don't want it. Why do you persist in keeping alive a fable?"

Mr. Melon never does respond to my query. He excuses himself by saying that he has another meeting and leaves my question forever unanswered. I never know whether it is the superintendent, the program administrators, or someone in the state capitol who terminates developmental therapy at Red Wing.

At last the day comes for my retirement party. My supervisor, Mr. Cunningham, sends a memo throughout the institution inviting all staff to come to bid me farewell. I worry that no one will come. But lo and behold, 94 of 750 staff attend. Some even congratulate me for proving that profoundly retarded children can learn. All sign my guest book, a notebook covered with red and white velvet which one of the teachers creates. I keep it as one of my treasured souvenirs.

I have spent almost twenty years at the Red Wing Institute and in the town of Red Wing. This means that most of my professional career has been devoted to training profoundly retarded persons and their care-givers. These years have given me crucial teaching on my journey into personhood. I have experienced scorn and jealousy from my colleagues as well as prolonged anger and depression because my department—then contributing to new knowledge about profoundly retarded individuals—was destroyed. And I have known great grief as I watched Mother's pain and gradual deterioration and worried over Belinda's illnesses and unhappiness.

I have also experienced the closeness and love of a small church. I have felt the joy of owning a home and supporting myself, caring for loved ones, having good neighbors, and making lifelong friends. Although frustrating at times, my twenty years at Red Wing have been full indeed.

Throughout the ups and downs of these years, I have known the comforting presence of my many spirit guides. In their human forms, they have visited in the daytime and have come after supper to dispel the evening's loneliness. At times, the Great Spirit himself has come in the aloneness of my den and the silence of the night to give me his peace. With this gift has come the courage to continue my journey.

10

My Journey, a Path to Faith

Change eventually comes. In the first week of January 1990, my brother, David, flies west and rents a car to drive Belinda and me to a retirement community called "the Entrance." Located in a college town in Iowa, it is affiliated with the United Church of Christ. In our own apartment, Belinda and I each have a bedroom and bath, and I have room for my IBM computer and for the remnant of my book collection. The Entrance's automatic doors and convenient curb cuts along four blocks give me the long-wanted freedom to shop in town and to go to church alone.

But Belinda is very unhappy because she misses her friends in Red Wing. Some residents of our new community do not know how to relate to her, and she begins again to express her fear and anger about our move in pseudo-seizures and various pains. Two years pass before she tells me, "Dr. Webb, I really like it here!" Although Belinda still suffers from a too-ready susceptibility to any virus which is currently in the neighborhood, she is now happily in the community's daycare program.

I, too, am haunted by a familiar problem. I am again receiving quizzical looks from my new neighbors who have never known a person with c.p. and so react very cautiously to my appearance and speech. My difficult communication is also an obstacle to making friends with persons who are hard of hearing. Seeking to be polite and yet avoid embarrassment, these people just turn away from me. In moments of great stress, the harder I try to speak plainly, the more jumbled my speech becomes. This causes deep frustration in me and great embarrassment to my listener.

Intellectually, I know that strangers who are unfamiliar with me may have one of three reactions. Their appraisal of my capabilities will be sympathetically down-to-earth, unrealistically optimistic, or unduly pessimistic. The understanding stranger readily ignores my abnormal speech, appearance, and movements and accepts me as an intelligent and responsible human being. On the other hand, the overoptimistic observer may conceal anxiety by placing me on a pedestal, far beyond anyone's reach and remark, "Oh, my dear Ruth, I don't see how you can go to work every morning with your handicap!"

The put-down reaction comes when "superior" observers dismiss me with a humiliating pat on my head. Then I hear the words, "Oh, you poor child. What a shame you are handicapped!"

Then my anger flares to a white heat! No other signal arouses my ire so quickly and so profoundly as to be treated like a child or a know-nothing. An uncontrollable reflex action is activated when my idea of myself, i.e. my self-concept, is threatened by word, deed, or attitude of those around me. I am not proud of this emotional reaction but cannot deny it is mine. It reflects the irrepressible part of me that insists on being recognized as a person.

Many of my struggles with such put-downs have come because I have tried to become a person in fact as well as in reputation. It has always cut me to the quick when my outward appearance, speech, and movements are taken as true reflection of my inner being.

Now in my retirement, I wonder how to deal with these new put-downs from well-meaning strangers. Once again, I have to prove that I am a person and not just a collection of strange sounds and movements.

While I do make friends with some wonderful people, I am un-happy and do not quite know why. I recognize that this is the be-ginning of the last period of my life. Perhaps this is the time to appraise the progress I have made on my journey into personhood. I begin to review my life and to ask these crucial questions.

Have I acquired the status of personhood, not only in my own eyes, but also in the opinion of friends as well as strangers? Will I be remembered as a contributing and responsible person or as a helpless cripple with awkward movements, hard-to-understand speech, and no ability to make decisions?

The longer I explore this question, the more alone I feel. There seems no one here whom I can trust to understand my fear that I have not become a real person. Dreary days grow into endless weeks. Fears, angers, unfulfilled hopes, and unresolved guilts dis-turb my sleep and sap my daytime energy.

There are days when I feel angry all over again about the breakup of my Developmental Therapy Department. Although my research and training techniques to help severely and profoundly retarded persons were widely distributed, they are now all lost because of jealous colleagues and my own administrative mistakes. My rage can only be expended on myself. Because I cannot release this an-ger, either verbally or physically, hot rage sweeps through me again and again. My stomach aches and I cannot sleep.

I keep remembering how my mother suffered from shingles and how I never found a doctor to alleviate her itching, burning pain. With the memory of her illness comes an additional guilt: Mother mournfully lamented that the room I had built for her was too small.

One night I realize that my greatest anger is against God for my cerebral palsy. Created by countless frustrations throughout my childhood by my physical inability to achieve what my mind desired, I cast my accumulated wrath on the Great Spirit. As foaming waves beat uselessly against the unyielding rocks, so I throw my angry self again and again against my Creator.

Now loneliness pervades my entire being. I am convinced that there is no one in the world who can enter my dark shroud. Even God has abandoned me. I am ready to give up. I even consider suicide.

I begin to weep in my study when Belinda is not home. I cannot wait long for expected events without crying. I am very ashamed that I have to cry when I get angry. My inner being cries out, Can't my injured brain let me wait? Do I have to weep when I am angry? Do I as an adult bear responsibility for my angry tears, or is my lack of control a result of my injured brain?

I feel these questions must be answered if my journey is to be completed successfully. To advance into personhood, I must assume responsibility for my emotions. But if my behavior is really caused by brain mechanisms, am I to blame when I lose emotional control? In calm minutes, I assume responsibility for my actions, but in the heat of anger, I blame my birth injury for my misbehavior. For me this is a never-ending argument between the prosecuting and defense attorneys within me.

At this point a remarkable spirit guide comes to lead me out of this slough of despondence. Little do I realize that my entire journey into personhood and my path to faith will acquire new meanings under her guidance. With expert deftness, she cuts to the heart of my troubles and declares that I am not only angry but also afraid. "Why?" she asks and leaves me to find the answer.

Eventually I solve the puzzle and recognize that my deep fear and anger originate from rejection by the "big girls" at the New England Institute of Learning. I have never forgiven my tormentors, and so over the years, fear has added its paralysis to the terrible anger aroused by my cerebral palsy. I now realize that I have suffered from these emotional wounds all through my learning and working careers. With the help of my counselor spirit, I review the hurts of the past and my anger and fear gradually recede. It takes a long time before my depression and recrimination diminish.

A perplexing question persists in my mind. Why am I brain-injured and subject to perseverating thoughts? My "logical" answer to the query goes like this: Every happening has a cause; because my brain did not receive sufficient oxygen during my twenty-nine-hour birth, it did not develop in the same way as in an uninjured child, and so when I am upset, thoughts occur over and over in my brain. My long birth changed forever the way my brain and body operate.

Why was my birth prolonged? Was it because the doctor was late in arriving or was it God's will? Neither explanation absolves me of any responsibility for my uncontrolled anger. I finally ask myself, Is it my task to find the answer to this riddle?

Some nights I lie awake for many hours thinking of this problem. Words without voice begin to reverberate in my mind. They tell me that I am loved as I am and that the Great Spirit has a purpose for me about which he will tell me when I am ready.

One particular night, the wordless voice whispers in my mind, "Ruth, don't be afraid of your anger. It covers up your fear of rejection. You must face this fear to dissolve it. When you are no longer afraid, you will no longer be angry."

The next morning as I awake I hear these words, "Ruth, you must give up being angry at the Great Spirit and at yourself as well as at the persons who have wronged you. When you stop pouring vengeance into your body, you will be freed from the bonds of anger. Forgiving yourself also prepares your heart to receive God's love."

A week later the voice without words speaks again. "Ruth, your loneliness may be used to reach toward God or you may allow it to drag you into depression. Then it may prevent you from successfully completing your journey. Invoking God's presence with prayer such

as 'Jesus, help me!' will disperse loneliness and strengthen your relationship with God."

Then suddenly, these words come into my mind. "Ruth, you have
a special mission from the Lord, the Great Spirit. Your mission is
similar to that of the man born blind about whom John, the gospel
writer, wrote. You, too, are asked to reflect God's glory in your disabled body. Without knowing your assignment, you have faithfully
pursued this mission by helping everyone you met on your journey.
The time has now come for you to pursue this mission actively. To
do this, you need to review the battles you have won. Remember,
with each victory, you have taken another step on your journey
into personhood."

During the next several months, I often awake around four
o'clock in the morning and watch as a panorama of triumphal
scenes passes rapidly through my mind. First, I am taking my first
solo walk at the Citizens' Rehabilitation Institute, tense with
fright. I feel great triumph when I finally reach Fran, my joyfully
weeping therapist, after crossing the empty and scary hall all alone.
Next I remember my trip down the aisle in my motor chair to be
hooded as a new Ph.D. Again I am living alone in my apartment
and taking care of my dog, Ginger, at the Institute for Better
Speech. Then I am helping clients in White Horse find jobs. In the
next moment I am planning a developmental therapy program for
little Charlie at Red Wing.

These glimpses of the past remind me that my twenty-year career
achievements have truly been steps forward on my journey into
personhood. Each step has been taken with the help of the caring
persons who have been my spirit guides.

When I recall the many spirit guides who have come to me in the
right way and at the right time, crucial coincidences, perhaps arranged by spirit guides, come to mind. If my mother had not been
so persistent that I do my exercises and if she had not been a teacher
who revered education, I may not have learned to read and to walk.
It was my dad's deferred desire for a Ph.D. that made him urge me

to seek a doctorate. And if the chancellor of Syracuse University had not spoken at my Drew commencement, I would have never been admitted to that university or been prepared for Dr. Walt's Ph.D. program at the University of Illinois.

My first job in the vocational workshop in White Horse, Wisconsin, came because of my friendship with Bob Linch, a fellow c.p. If I had not met Anna on my first visit to Red Wing, I may not have had a career at Red Wing. When frustrations at home and on the job threatened to overwhelm me, I would have despaired if psychotherapist Dorothy had not helped me regain my emotional balance.

Many nights I hear this whisper, "I am always with you. As Joe Bishop told you long ago, my help will always come to you when you need me. The review of your life has shown you our loving care throughout your life."

As I ponder these scenes throughout many days and weeks, I begin to catch a vision. Jesus Christ, the Son of the Great Spirit, has been the Chief Spirit Guide on my lifelong journey into personhood. I have not searched for Him as much as He has guided me. He has indeed lived in my struggles to be a person. I know He has always been my Chief Spirit Guide because Jesus has shown Himself to me on many occasions in many different ways.

I can never forget these times: The scene in the Norman Chapel at Silver Bay CFO when a light fell upon my friend the Rev. Chet and me as we prayed; again that light shone around world literacy expert Dr. Frank Laubach as he invoked God's blessing on the communion bread; it was in the same chapel that the wind of the Holy Spirit blew over us in response to Tommy Tyson's prayer.

I remember walking down the sandy hill alone at my aunt's home on Martha's Vineyard, supported by an unseen presence and the healing, life-changing "soup" which flooded my being when Agnes Sanford, Joe Bishop, and I encountered God. I will always give thanks for Carola, who first made me realize that God's love is always with me.

But even with these assurances, there still are times when I doubt my progress into personhood. Then I wonder, Am I now a full-fledged person not only in the opinion of others but also in my own? Have I completely dispelled my rage over my cerebral palsy? My destroyed career? Do I respond to ridiculing strangers with understanding instead of anger? Am I reconciled to my loneliness? These questions remain to be answered.

I now realize my ongoing journey into personhood has led me along the path of faith. My search for integrity as a person has not only brought yearned-for opportunities to give and receive love. In that giving and receiving, my grandfather's prediction has come true. I have come to know the Son of the Great Spirit.

When the time comes to take my blanket "off the loom," I trust my Chief Guide and His Father, the Great Spirit, will see beauty in its patterns despite the many knots and tangles on the underside. For His promise, "My grace is sufficient for you," gives me courage to complete the pattern He is helping me weave.

Singular Lives